Davis's Notes

Your Handheld Clinical Companions

e vital clinical information you need!

PAA-supportive, wipe-free, waterproof,
sable patient assessment tools and worksheets
rtable, indispensable, pocket-sized tools for safe
d effective health care delivery

ing Notes: Medical Insurance Pocket Guide
ides students and practicing Medical Assistants
an easy-to-understand medical billing and
ng reference. Formatted in text, tables, and
s to help users quickly and accurately find
rmation for immediate use.

Coding Notes—Coding and billing made easy!

Look for our other Davis's Notes titles

RNotes® • MedSurg Notes • NutriNotes • MedNotes • LPN Notes
MA Notes: Medical Assistant's Pocket Guide
IV Therapy Notes: Nurse's Clinical Pocket Guide
LabNotes: Guide to Lab & Diagnostic Tests
ECG Notes: Interpretation and Management Guide

Visit us at www.FADavis.com

F.A. Davis Company
Independent Publishers Since 1879

ISBN 10: 0-8036-1493-4
ISBN 13: 978-0-8036-1493-2

9 780803 614932

Inches   Centimeters

F. A. Davis Company

Always at your side...

Coding
Notes

Medical Insurance Pocket Guide

Alice Anne Andress

Waterproof and Reusable

Includes...
- ✔ Wipe-Free Forms
- ✔ Submitting Claims
- ✔ Understanding Insurance Carriers
- ✔ CPT, ICD-9-CM, and HCPCS Coding
- ✔ Modifiers

- ✔ Code Changes from ICD-9 to ICD-10
- ✔ Documentation
- ✔ Medical Decision Matrix
- ✔ Specialty Coding Billing Guidelines for PAs and NPs Too!

Contacts • Phone/E-Mail

Name:	
Ph:	e-mail:

Name:	
Ph:	e-mail:

Name:	
Ph:	e-mail:

Name:	
Ph:	e-mail:

Name:	
Ph:	e-mail:

Name:	
Ph:	e-mail:

Name:	
Ph:	e-mail:

Name:	
Ph:	e-mail:

Name:	
Ph:	e-mail:

Name:	
Ph:	e-mail:

Name:	
Ph:	e-mail:

Name:	
Ph:	e-mail:

Name:	
Ph:	e-mail:

Coding
Notes

Medical Insurance Pocket Guide

Alice Anne Andress, CCS-P, CCP

Purchase additional copies of this book at your health science bookstore or directly from F. A. Davis by shopping online at www.fadavis.com or by calling 800-323-3555 (US) or 800-665-1148 (CAN)

A Davis's Notes Book

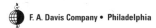

F. A. Davis Company • Philadelphia

F. A. Davis Company
1915 Arch Street
Philadelphia, PA 19103
www.fadavis.com

Printed in China by Imago

Last digit indicates print number: 10 9 8 7 6 5 4 3 2 1

Acquisition Editor: Andy McPhee
Developmental Editor: Melissa Reed
Manager of Art & Design: Carolyn O'Brien
Reviewers: Darlene Kaye Acton, CMA; Korene Silvestri Atkins, MA, RHIA, CCS, CPC, CPC-H; Kay E. Biggs, BS, CMA; Ursula Cole, RHE, MAED, BAED; Willa Davis, CMBS, CPT; Liza Strickland Kerssemakers, CPC; Michelle Shipley, RRA, CCS; Barbara Tietsort, MED

Current Procedural Terminology (CPT) is copyright 2005 American Medical Association. All Rights Reserved. No fee schedules, basic units, relative values, or related listings are included in CPT. The AMA assumes no liability for the data contained herein. Applicable FARS/DFARS restrictions apply to government use.

CPT® is a trademark of the American Medical Association.

As new scientific information becomes available through basic and clinical research, recommended treatments and drug therapies undergo changes. The author(s) and publisher have done everything possible to make this book accurate, up to date, and in accord with accepted standards at the time of publication. The author(s), editors, and publisher are not responsible for errors or omissions or for consequences from application of the book, and make no warranty, expressed or implied, in regard to the contents of the book. Any practice described in this book should be applied by the reader in accordance with professional standards of care used in regard to the unique circumstances that may apply in each situation. The reader is advised always to check product information (package inserts) before administering any drug. Caution is especially urged when using new or infrequently ordered drugs.

Rosihy as amend

Place $2\frac{7}{8} \times 2\frac{7}{8}$ **Sticky Notes** here
For a convenient and refillable note pad

✓ **HIPAA Compliant**
✓ **OSHA Compliant**

**Waterproof and Reusable
Wipe-Free Pages**

**Write directly onto any page of *Coding Notes*
with a ballpoint pen. Wipe old entries off with
an alcohol pad and reuse.**

| GEN EVAL | MGMT SURG | ANES RAD | PATHOL | MED | ICD-9-CM | MOD/HCPCS | TOOLS |

General Billing and Insurance Guidelines
Patient Registration Form

The patient registration form is one of the most important forms in a medical practice. It contains all necessary information required for billing for services and procedures. This form should be updated yearly. Patient information should be reviewed and verified at each patient encounter to ensure that the practice has the most current and accurate information on file.

Each item on the form should be verified by asking the patient, "Do you still live at ...." instead of using a general statement such as "Has anything changed since your last visit?"

A copy of the patient's health insurance card, both front and back, should be copied during each visit.

This form should contain the following information:

Data	Reason
Date	Required for billing purposes
Patient's name	Required for billing purposes
Patient's address	Required for billing purposes
Patient's phone number	Required for billing purposes and to contact patient regarding appointments and testing results
Patient's date of birth	Required for billing purposes
Patient age	Required for billing purposes
Patient's Social Security number	Required for patient identification purposes only
Guarantor's name, address, and phone number if patient is not guarantor	Required for billing purposes
Employer's name, address, and phone number	Required for billing purposes or if patient needs to be contacted during working hours

(Continued text on following page)

Data	Reason
Spouse's name	May be required for billing purposes
Spouse's employer's name, address, and phone number	May be required for billing purposes or if spouse needs to be contacted during working hours
Insurance company name, address, and phone number	Required for billing purposes
Insurance identification and group numbers	Required for billing purposes
Person to be notified in case of emergency	Required in case of emergency
Referred by	Required for billing and quality of care purposes
Patient signature	Required for billing purposes
Some forms will contain the following:	
List of current medications	For clinical reasons
Past illnesses/surgeries	
Allergies	

Review this form for completeness as this information is critical to the billing process. Any missing information should be completed by asking the patient questions.

There are some key areas to look for that may be "tell-tale" for nonpaying patients. These areas are:

- Incomplete information on the form
- Questionable employment information
- No phone number
- Post office box listed instead of a street address
- Motel address
- No insurance information
- No referral information

A potential nonpaying patient may sometimes be identified by items on the above list.

If any of the above elements exist, extra care should be taken to obtain accurate and complete information.

Patient Encounter Form

One of the most important factors in medical billing is an accurate form. This form has many names: patient encounter form, superbill, fee slip, charge slip, billing form, etc. This form is used to communicate the patient visit charges to the billing personnel. All information on this form must be accurate and complete and contain the following data:

- Patient's name
- Patient's address
- Patient's home phone number
- Patient's account number/medical record number
- Guarantor's name
- Patient/guarantor's insurance company and identification number
- Date of service
- Patient's date of birth
- Provider name
- Diagnosis section
- CPT code section
- Space for next appointment
- Space for provider to complete with any studies that may need to be ordered

This form must be reviewed and updated twice a year when the codes are updated. Deleted codes, new codes, and revised codes should be updated when necessary.

Life Cycle of an Insurance Form

New Patient, Office

A new patient is one who has not been seen by the physician or any physician in that specialty group within the last 3 years. These visits are reported using codes 99201–99205. Detailed information regarding these codes can be found in Tab 2.

*Current Procedural Terminology © 2006 American Medical Association, All Rights Reserved.

The steps involved in an office visit for a new patient are:

Step 1	Patient information
The patient arrives at the office. The patient is either interviewed or completes a patient registration form to obtain information listed to the right. If the patient registration form is not completed in its entirety, the office staff should question the patient in order to obtain all the necessary information. Some offices will have the patient complete a history form as well.	Name
	Address
	Phone number
	Place of employment
	Spouse name, if applicable
	Emergency contact info
	Allergies
	Reason for visit
	Type of insurance
	Address of insurance
	Sign a record release form, if applicable

OR

Step 1	Patient information
The patient calls the office to make an appointment. Information is collected via the phone call to obtain the data as listed to the right. Patient is asked to bring his/her insurance card to the office visit.	Name
	Address
	Phone number
	Place of employment
	Spouse name, if applicable
	Emergency contact info
	Allergies
	Reason for visit
	Type of insurance
	Address of insurance

Step 2	Insurance
The patient arrives at the office with his/her insurance card.	Patient registration form is completed.
	Both sides of the insurance card are copied.
	This copy is placed in the patient's chart.
	All patients with insurance must sign an authorization of benefits form to allow the practice to release information necessary for payment of the claim and to request that payment be made directly to the physician practice.
	Depending on insurance, verification of coverage may be necessary.
	If this is a specialty office and the patient has a managed care plan, a referral is necessary for treatment.
	Most managed care plans have co-pays, which must be paid at the time of the visit.
	If the patient has Medicare, a deductible must be met at the beginning of each calendar year.
	If the patient has Medicaid or other insurances, there may be deductibles and co-pays that are necessary to be paid. This information can be found on the insurance card.
	If the patient is a child, be aware of the birthday rule. If both parents carry insurance, the child will be covered under the parent whose birthday is first in a calendar year.

(Continued text on following page)

Step 3	Create the chart
A patient chart is created with the forms listed to the right.	Place patient registration form and copy of insurance card in chart.
	Place all other authorization forms in the chart.
	Any forms used by the practice to record clinical information, such as medication logs, progress note forms, office visit templates, history forms, problem lists, etc.
	Apply appropriate labels to the chart, such as type of insurance, year of visit, alphabetized labels indicating the patient name for faster filing.

Step 4	Data entry

A patient account is created in the computer using the following information from the patient registration and insurance card.

Step 5	Generate a patient encounter form
A patient encounter form is generated and placed on the front of the patient's chart. This document becomes the source of information for billing. This document has many names, some of which you can see in the column to the right.	Fee slip
	Superbill
	Charge slip
	Billing form
	Charge capture form

The patient is seen by the physician and is discharged from that office visit.

Established Patient, Office

An established patient is one who has been seen by the physician within the last 3 years. These visits are reported using codes 99211–99215. Detailed information regarding these codes can be found in Tab 2.

The steps involved in an office visit for an established patient are:

Step 1	Scheduling of appointment

The patient either schedules a follow-up appointment while at the office or calls the office for an appointment.

Step 2	Preauthorization of services or procedures

If the physician is a specialist, the staff must check the preauthorization to be sure it has not expired. If the referral has expired, it will be necessary to obtain a new form from the primary care physician. Most physician offices submit referrals electronically.

Step 3	Review and update patient registration form

Be sure all information listed on the patient registration form is accurate and complete. These forms should be completely updated yearly; however, at each patient visit, the staff should inquire as to any changes that may have occurred in the patient's insurance, address, employment, etc.

Step 4	Collect co-pays and deductibles

All co-pays should be collected at the time of patient check-in. For Medicare patients, deductibles are not collected at the time of the service. Medicare is billed, and any deductible still due is deducted from the physician payment. This is stated on the Explanation of Medicare Benefits. The patient is then billed for the deductible amount.

(Continued text on following page)

Step 5	Generate a patient encounter form
A patient encounter form is generated and placed on the front of the patient's chart. This document becomes the source of information for billing. This document has many names, some of which are in the column to the right.	Fee slip
	Superbill
	Charge slip
	Billing form
	Charge capture form

The purpose of the patient encounter form is to communicate charges (services and procedures the patient received) and diagnoses to the billing department. This form is also used to inform the staff of any diagnostic studies that are to be ordered and to indicate any follow-up appointments that may be necessary. The patient is seen by the physician and is discharged from that office visit.

Patient Discharge	
Step 1	**Charges**
Physician practice has check-out procedures.	The patient charges are totaled on the patient encounter form.
Step 2	**Posting**
	The patient charges are posted to the patient's account in the computer system.
Step 3	**Payment**
Patient's financials	If no insurance, the patient is expected to pay at the time of the service.

Step 3	Payment
	If the patient has a co-pay that has not been collected during check-in, the patient is expected to pay at discharge.
	If the patient has insurance that does not cover office visits, the patient is expected to pay at the time of service.
	Any payment made is then posted to the patient's account.

The purpose of the CMS 1500 claim form is to create a standard for collecting Medicare information. The most common claim denials, based on the claim form, are the result of incomplete or inaccurate diagnosis codes (Box 21) and incorrect place of service codes (Box 24b). The CMS 1500 Form information is complete, accurate, and ready for submission when all items in the table below have been completed.

Step 4	Generate insurance form (CMS 1500 Form)

Step 5	Attachments
For filing paper claims only	Copy and staple any attachments that are necessary to the form. If no attachments are necessary, form can be sent electronically.
	Attachments are needed if there is a concurrent care situation, if an unusual service or procedure was performed.

Step 6	Signature, patient
Signatures are an important part of the form.	The patient must sign the form if the paper form is being sent.
	For claims where the patient has signed an authorization form, the phrase "SOF" or "signature on file" can print in box 12.

(Continued text on following page)

Step 6	Signature, patient
	If the form is being submitted electronically, "SOF" or "signature on file" can print in box 12.
	When an illiterate or physically handicapped patient signs by a mark (X), a witness must enter his or her name and address next to the mark on the form.
	A representative may sign the form on the patient's behalf if the patient is physically or mentally unable to sign. When this occurs, the signature line must indicate the patient's name followed by the word "by", the representative's name, address, relationship to the patient, and the reason the patient cannot sign.
	If there is no signature, the claim will not be transferred automatically to Medigap.
Step 6a	**Signature, provider**
Signatures are an important part of the form.	The claim must be signed by the provider or an authorized representative if the form is being provided on paper.
	No signature is necessary if the form is being sent electronically.
	A signature stamp may be used if the provider's name is typed below.
Step 7	**Insurance tracking**
Submitted claims should be tracked.	If the claim is manually produced (paper), an insurance log must be kept, with information such as the patient name, amount of claim, insurance carrier, and date submitted.
	If the claim is submitted electronically, the computer will provide the practice with a report.

Step 8	Submit claim
	Either mail or submit the form electronically.
	Forms should be submitted daily for better cash flow.
	When submitting a form electronically, run a presubmission report to identify any errors that may cause denials and correct them before submittal.

Step 9	Check is mailed
A check along with an explanation of benefits (EOB) is mailed to the provider if the provider is participating.	Information is taken from the EOB and posted to the patient's account.
	Any claim denials must thoroughly reviewed, corrected, and resubmitted if possible.
	Automatic rebilling of claims to the carrier without investigation and analysis of the claim can result in duplicate claims and duplicate payments. This can be construed as fraudulent billing.

Preauthorization/Precertification

Preauthorization:
Some insurance carriers require permission to perform a service or procedure before it is done. This preauthorization identifies whether the insurance program will allow the service or procedure to be performed based on the medical necessity information provided.

Precertification:
Identifies whether the service or procedure is covered under the patient's insurance plan. Precertification is not based on the medical necessity of the procedure but on whether the patient has coverage.

Although proper steps have been taken to obtain preauthorization/precertification, there is no guarantee that services will be covered.

Completion of a CMS 1500 Form

CMS Areas	Completion Instructions
Box 1: Type of insurance	Medicare, Medicaid, Champus/Tricare, group health plan, FECA/black lung, other
Box 1a: Insured's ID number	Contains the patient's health insurance number
Box 2: Patient name	Enter patient's name exactly as it is on the insurance card
	Address, phone number
	Do not leave a space between a prefix and a name
	For hyphenated names, capitalize both names and separate by a hyphen
	Leave a space between the last name and a suffix
Box 3: Patient's date of birth and sex	Enter date of birth using two digits for the month, two for the day, and four for the year: MM/DD/YYYY
	Check the box that indicates the sex of the patient; the sex of the patient must be valid for the diagnosis of the patient
Box 4: Insured's name	For Medicare: Enter the name of the insured person only if that person's insurance is primary to Medicare; if Medicare is primary, leave it blank
Box 5: Patient's address	Enter the complete mailing address and telephone number
	If the patient lives in a nursing home, list the nursing home address as the patient's
	Do not place punctuation in a city name that contains an abbreviation

CMS Areas	Completion Instructions
Box 6: Patient relationship to the insured	This relationship is to the primary insured; choices are self, spouse, child, other
	Complete this box only if Box 4 is completed; otherwise leave it blank
Box 7: Insured's address	Complete this box only if Box 4 is completed; otherwise leave it blank
Box 8: Patient's status	Indicate the patient's marital status and employment or student status
	The choices for marital status are single, married, other
	The choices for employment are employed, full-time student, part-time student
Box 9: Other insured's name	Enter the name of the insured person who is enrolled in a Medigap policy if the name is different from the name shown in Box 2; enter the word "same" if it is the same
Box 10: Is patient's condition related to:	If the patient's condition is related to employment, an automobile accident, or some other accident
	This information is used for coordination of benefits
	If the patient's condition is not related to any of these, place an X in the "No" box for each item
Box 11: Insured's Policy Group or FECA number	
Box 11a: Insured's date of birth	Date of birth and sex of the individual who carries the insurance
Box 11b: Emp-loyer's name	Name of the employer of the individual who carriers the insurance
Box 11c: Insurance plan name or program name	Name of insurance plan of the individual who carriers the insurance

(Continued text on following page)

GEN
EVAL

CMS Areas	Completion Instructions
Box 11d: Is there another health benefit plan?	Answer whether there is a secondary insurance
Box 12: Patient's or authorized person's signature	Enter the signature of the patient or the patient's representative and the date; this signature allows for the release of information necessary to process the claim
Box 13: Medigap benefits authorization	The insured's signature must be entered in this block
Box 14: Date of current illness, injury, or pregnancy	Enter the date of the current illness (first symptom), injury (accident), or pregnancy (last menstrual period)
	If an accident date is entered, complete Box 10b or 10c
	For chiropractic services, enter the date of the initiation of the course of treatment and the x-ray date in Box 19
Box 15: If patient has had same or similar illness	Do not complete this box for Medicare patients
	For all other insurers, the date should match the date or be later than the date entered in Box 24a
Box 16: Dates patient unable to work	This block provides the dates that the patient was employed but unable to work
	This field MUST be completed for all Workers Compensation claims
Box 17: Name of referring physician	Enter the name of the physician who requested the service
Box 17a: ID number of referring physician	Enter the UPIN number of the referring physician; if the referring physician does not have a UPIN number, a surrogate number may be used

CMS Areas	Completion Instructions
Box 18: Hospitaliza-tion dates related to current services	Enter the admission and discharge dates
	If the services were rendered in a facility other than the patient's home or a physician's office, provide the name and address of that facility in Box 32
Box 19: Reserved for local use	Leave box blank
Box 20: Outside diagnostic services	Place a "Yes" in the box when a provider (other than the provider billing for the service) performed the diagnostic test; when "Yes" is checked, Box 32 must be completed
	Enter the purchase price of the tests in the charges column; show the dollars and cents, omitting the dollar sign
Box 21: Diagnosis or nature of illness or injury	Enter the ICD-9-CM code for the diagnoses, conditions, problems, or other reasons for the visit
	Report at least one diagnosis per claim
	Only four diagnosis codes can be submitted
Box 22: Medicaid resubmission	Enter the codes and original Medicaid reference number of a Medicaid claim
	This area must be completed when resubmitting a claim to Medicaid
Box 23: Prior authori-zation number	Enter the number assigned by the peer review organization
	For laboratory services performed by a physician office laboratory (POL), enter the 10-digit CLIA certification number

(Continued text on following page)

CMS Areas	Completion Instructions
Box 24a: Date(s) of service	Enter the beginning and end date of service for the entire period reflected by the procedure code
Box 24b: Place of service	Enter the appropriate two-digit place of service code; see Tab 8: Tools
Box 24c: Type of service	Enter the code describing the type of service rendered
	This should not be completed when the claim is Medicare
Box 24d: Procedures, service, or supplies	Enter the appropriate CPT or HCPCS code for the procedures, service, or supply
Box 24e: Diagnosis code	Enter the appropriate diagnosis code that is linked to the procedures, service, or supply
Box 24f: Charges	Enter the amount charged by the physician for each of the services or procedures listed on the claim
	Do not bill a flat fee for multiple dates of service
Box 24g: Days or units	Enter the number of days or units of procedures, services, or supplies listed in Box 24d
Box 24h: EPSDT	Early periodic screening, diagnosis, and treatment services
	These services apply only to children who are 12 or younger and receive medical benefits through Medicaid
Box 24i: EMG	Enter a check if the service was rendered in a hospital emergency department
	Place of service "23" would be placed in Box 24b

CMS Areas	Completion Instructions
Box 24j: COB	When checked, indicates a coordination of benefits
Box 24k: Performing provider number	Enter the first two digits of the UPIN
Box 25: Federal tax ID number	Enter the Federal tax ID number or Social Security number of the physician or supplier
Box 26: Patient's account number	Enter the patient's account number; this will then be referenced on the Explanation of Benefits for easier posting of monies to the patient account
Box 27: Accept assignment?	Check "Yes" when the physician accepts assignment for the claim
Box 28: Total charge	Enter the total amount charged for all procedures, services, and supplies in Boxes 24f, lines 1 through 6
	Enter the dollars and cents without the dollar sign
Box 29: Amount paid	Enter the dollar amount paid toward the total cost of the service
Box 30: Balance due	Enter the dollar amount due after subtracting the amount paid
	If the claim is Medicare, leave this area blank.
Box 31: Signature of physician or supplier, including degrees or credentials	The provider or his or her representative must sign the provider's name
	A stamp may be used, but the provider's full name must be typed below the stamp
Box 32: Name and address of facility where services were rendered	If services were provided in a hospital, clinic, laboratory, or any facility other than the physician's office or the patient's home, this area must be completed

(Continued text on following page)

CMS Areas	Completion Instructions
	When the name and address are the same as in Box 33, place the word "Same" in this box
	If the physician provided services in a hospital (place of service 21, 22, 23), the Medicare provider number must also be placed in this box
Box 33: Physician's/ supplier's billing names, address, zip code, phone number	Enter the billing name, address, and telephone number of the physician or supplier who furnished the service

Place of Service Codes

When submitting a claim for reimbursement, a place of service code must be placed in Item 24b of a CMS 1500 form. Not all of the codes listed below are approved by all carriers. When performing a billing function, the carrier should be contacted to verify that the place of service code is valid.

Code	Type	Description
03	School	Service provided at school
04	Homeless shelter	Service provided at a shelter that serves as temporary housing for patient
05	Indian Health Service/ Freestanding facility	Service provided at a facility that is operated by the Indian Health Service where patients are not admitted
06	Indian Health Service/ Freestanding facility	Service provided at a facility that is operated by the Indian Health Service where patients are admitted as out- or inpatients

Code	Type	Description
07	Tribal 638 freestanding facility	Service is provided at a facility that is operated by the Indian Health Service under a 638 agreement, which provides diagnostic, therapeutic, and rehabilitation services to those who are not admitted
08	Tribal 638 freestanding facility	Service is provided at a facility that is operated by the Indian Health Service under a 638 agreement, which provides diagnostic, therapeutic, and rehabilitation services to those who are admitted as out- or inpatients
11	Office	Service provided in office setting
12	Home	Service provided in the patient's or caregiver's home
13	Assisted-living facility	Service provided in a residential facility with self-contained living units that provides support 24 hours a day; this facility has the capacity to arrange for other services if needed
14	Group home	Service provided at a shared living residence where patients receive supervision and other services such as social, behavioral, and custodial
15	Mobile unit	Service provided at a facility that moves from place to place to provide preventive, screening, diagnostic, and treatment services

(Continued text on following page)

GEN EVAL

Code	Type	Description
20	Urgent care facility	Service provided at a facility, separate from a hospital emergency room (ER), where patients can be diagnosed and treated for illness or injury; these patients require immediate medical attention
21	Inpatient hospital	Service provided at a hospital
22	Outpatient hospital	Service provided at a portion of the hospital that provides diagnostic, therapeutic, and rehabilitation services to patients who do not require admission
23	Emergency Room—Hospital	Service provided at a hospital ER
24	Ambulatory surgical center	Service provided at a freestanding facility where surgical and diagnostic services are provided on an ambulatory basis; cannot be provided in a physician's office
25	Birthing center	Service provided at a facility, separate from a hospital or physician's office, where maternity facilities are available
26	Military treatment facility	Service provided at a facility operated by the Uniformed Services
31	Skilled nursing facility	Service provided at a facility that provides inpatient skilled nursing care
32	Nursing facility	Service provided at a facility that provides patients with skilled nursing care and related services

Code	Type	Description
33	Custodial care	Service provided at a facility that provides room and board and other assistance to patients on a long-term basis without a medical component
34	Hospice	Service provided at a facility, other than the patient's home, where palliative and supportive care for terminally ill is provided
41	Ambulance: land	A land vehicle equipped to provide transportation and life-saving care to patients
42	Ambulance: air/water	An air or water vehicle equipped to provide transportation and life saving care to patients
49	Independent clinic	Service provided at a clinic, **not** part of a hospital, that is organized and operated to provide preventive, diagnostic, therapeutic, rehabilitative, or palliative services to patients
50	Federally qualified health center	Service provided at a facility located in a medically underserved area that provides Medicare patients with preventive care under the direction of a physician
51	Inpatient psychiatric facility	Service at a facility that provides inpatient psychiatric care for the diagnosis and treatment of mental illness on a 24-hour basis

(Continued text on following page)

Code	Type	Description
52	Psychiatric facility: partial hospitalization	Service at a facility for the diagnosis and treatment of mental illness that provides a planned therapeutic program for patients who do not require full-time hospitalization but who need broader programs than do outpatients
53	Community mental health center	Service at a facility that provides outpatient services for children, elderly, individuals who are chronically ill, and residents of the center who were discharged from inpatient treatment, day treatment, partial hospitalization, screening for patients being considered for admission to state mental health facilities to determine the appropriateness of such admission, and consultation and education services
54	Intermediate care facility/mentally retarded	Service at a facility that provides health-related care and services above the level of custodial care to mentally retarded patients
55	Residential substance abuse treatment facility	Service at a facility that provides treatment for substance abuse to live-in residents who do not require acute medical care
56	Psychiatric residential treatment center	Service at a facility for psychiatric care that provides a total 24-hour therapeutically and professionally staffed group living and learning environment

Code	Type	Description
57	Nonresidential substance abuse treatment facility	Service at a facility that provides treatment for substance abuse on an ambulatory basis
60	Mass immunization center	Service at a facility where providers administer pneumococcal pneumonia and influenza vaccines and submit these services for billing; can be a public health center, pharmacy, or mall
61	Comprehensive inpatient rehabilitation facility	Service at a facility that provides comprehensive rehabilitation services under the supervision of a physician to inpatients with physical disabilities; services include physical therapy (PT), occupational therapy (OT), speech pathology, psychological services, and orthotics and prosthetics
62	Comprehensive outpatient rehabilitation facility	Service at a facility that provides comprehensive rehabilitation services under the supervision of a physician to outpatients with physical disabilities; services include PT, OT, speech pathology, psychological services, and orthotics and prosthetics
65	End-stage renal disease treatment facility	Service provided at a facility other than a hospital, which provides dialysis treatment, maintenance, and/or training
71	State or local public health clinic	Service at a facility maintained by the state or local health department that provides ambulatory primary care under the direction of a physician

(Continued text on following page)

Code	Type	Description
72	Rural health clinic	Service at a facility, which is in a certified rural underserved area, that provides ambulatory primary care under the direction of a physician
81	Independent laboratory	Service at an independent laboratory that is certified to perform diagnostic and/or clinical tests
99	Other place of service	Other place of service not identified

Claims Submission Issues

There are some common problems identified with claims submissions:

- Incorrect insurance number
- Incorrect physician UPIN number
- Submission to an incorrect carrier
- Incorrect diagnosis code (missing, incomplete)
- Patient's name, address, etc. as listed does not match insurance carrier records
- Gender of patient incorrect
- Incorrect date of service
- Incorrect place of service code
- Incorrect or missing modifier(s)
- Incorrect units billed
- Missing provider ID number
- Illegible claim form

Explanation of Benefits (EOB)

An EOB or remittance advice identifies which services, procedures, and/or supplies were paid and which were denied. All denials will contain a reason code that fully explains the reason for denial. An EOB contains the following information:

Components of an Explanation of Benefits

- Patient name
- Patient ID number or HIC number
- Claim processing ID number
- Provider name
- Date of service
- Procedure code
- Diagnosis code
- Allowable charge
- Submitted charge
- What portion is deductible and/or co-pay
- What is paid and to whom
- Patient responsibility amount
- If no payment, the reason code for the non-payment

EOBs will not be sent to providers who do not accept assignment on claims. This is prohibited by the Federal Privacy Act of 1974. In this case, the EOB will be sent to the patient. If an appeal is required on a non-assigned claim, the patient must provide the EOB along with a letter stating the provider is permitted to assist in the appeal. The EOBs should be reviewed periodically to assure that the provider is receiving accurate reimbursement.

Denial of Claims

There are some common denials identified with claims submissions. Below you will find a listing with a recommendation to follow.

Rejected claims	Recommendation
Claims are often rejected due to incorrect or invalid information (date of birth, transposed numbers, provider numbers, dates of service, incorrect gender, etc) submitted to the carrier.	Review all claim information for accuracy and completeness before submission. Correct all rejected claims and resubmit.

Delays in payment	Recommendation
Delay can result due to claim being "in process," where the carrier is awaiting additional information requested from the provider or beneficiary.	Correct claims quickly and resubmit so that cash flow is not interrupted. Claims that have been suspended awaiting information from the patient are more difficult to handle. Once the practice verifies that the delay lies with the patient, the practice should call the patient to suggest that the practice could help provide this information.

Service was not covered by insurance	Recommendation
Some services are not considered to be a covered service, e.g., hearing test, eyeglasses, preventive medicine, etc.	Send the patient a letter explaining that the claim was denied due to lack of coverage. This charge now becomes the patient's responsibility.

Service provided was for a pre-existing condition	Recommendation
Some services cannot be reimbursed as the patient has a pre-existing condition (a condition for which they have already obtained care).	When the patient presents to the office as a new patient, ask about any pre-existing conditions. When performing a service or procedure that may fall under that condition, always check with the carrier to see if a pre-existing clause exists. If so, discuss the charge with the patient to identify whether the patient wants to proceed, with the understanding that the patient will have to pay.
Deductible was not met	**Recommendation**
The patient is responsible for a certain dollar amount of deductible each year. Payment cannot be made until that deductible is met.	Ask the patient on arrival whether he or she has seen any other physicians since January 1 of that calendar year. This may provide some insight into what may have already been applied to the deductible. The best practice is to submit the bill to the insurance carrier and to review the EOB/remittance advice to identify what dollar amount has been applied to the deductible. Once that figure is obtained, bill the patient for the deductible amount.

Check Verification

A personal check is the most common form of payment in a medical office. Important facts regarding checks:

- Always check the name and address on a personal check against the patient's driver's license.
- On any suspicious or out-of-town check, call the bank to verify that the funds are available. It is a good practice not to accept out-of-town checks; however, some practices are located in resort areas where out-of-town checks are common. In this case, attempt to have the patient pay by credit/debit card.
- Do not accept third-party checks.
- Do not cash checks over the amount due to give the patient cash back.
- Do not accept a check in which the patient has inscribed "payment in full" on the check. Once this check is cashed, it could be argued that no additional payment is needed.
- Be sure the check is signed. If the unsigned check is from an established patient and merely an oversight, the practice should try to reach the patient to request she or he stop by to sign the check. If it is difficult for the patient to return to sign the check, the check can be handled in the following manner:
- Write the word "over" on the signature line of the check.
- On the back of the check in the endorsement area, write "Lack of signature guaranteed," the practice's name, and the writer's own name and title. This tells the bank that the practice will accept the loss in such a case where the patient would not honor the check.

*Some offices charge an additional administrative fee for returned checks. This amount would also have to be included in the letter.

Returned Checks

The most common reason for a check to be returned is for nonsufficient funds (NSF).* When this occurs, do the following:

- Redeposit the check, or call the patient to see if the check can be redeposited. Most banks will allow a redeposit one time.

- If the check cannot be redeposited, ask the patient how he or she would like to cover this outstanding balance: credit card, debit, cash, etc.
- If the check is returned after a second deposit, call the patient and ask how he or she intends to resolve this matter. If this phone call becomes difficult, send a letter demanding payment. This letter should include the following information:
- Check date
- Check number
- The bank on which it was drawn
- The name of the person who wrote the check
- The name of the person to whom the check was payable
- The amount of the check
- The number of days the patient has to correct the matter

*Some offices charge an additional administrative fee for returned checks. This amount would also have to be included in the letter.

Financial Hardship

When patients have true financial problems and inability to pay, a reasonable attempt must be made to collect the fee. A reasonable attempt to collect would be demonstrated by the following:

- Any collection process used to collect an amount from a non-Medicare patient
- Patient statements sent to either the patient or the guarantor
- Collection letters or telephone calls in an effort to collect payment; all telephone calls should be documented to create a paper trail

Once it has been determined that the patient is a true hardship case, the provider must determine the patient's ability to pay through a review of additional information requested from the patient.

- Request a copy of the patient's tax form from the previous year or a copy of the W-2 or statement of earnings from the Social Security Administration
- Some practices have developed financial determination forms for the patient to complete

Unpaid Claims

An old trial balance report should be obtained from the practice's computer. This report should be used to follow up on all unpaid claims. This report can be run by the insurance carrier or as one general report.

Step 1

Run computer-generated Aged Trial Balance report. The report can be generated with the following parameters:

- By insurance carrier
- By provider
- By codes
- By dollar amount
- By practice (includes all providers, all codes, all carriers)

Step 2

Begin follow-up by starting with the largest dollar amount listed and continue through the smallest amount

Step 3a

If no EOB was received, call carrier to obtain status of claim

Step 3b

If EOB was received, review EOB to ascertain reason for the denial

Step 4a

If claim requires additional information from the provider, this should be completed and then resubmitted.

Step 4b

Follow up on denial reason code; correct error and resubmit

Step 5

Never resubmit a claim without proper investigation into why it was not paid

Insurance Commissioner

There is an insurance commissioner in each state where insurance problems can be reported for further action. Examples of some of these problems are:

- Delays in payment by third-party carriers
- Incorrect denial of claims
- Incorrect termination of a policy

Have information available when contacting the commissioner. Such information would be:

- Patient name, address, phone number
- Insured's name address, phone number
- Name of insurance company
- Policy number
- Problem

Collections

Statute of Limitations

Each state has a statute of limitations, which sets a time limit* on the maximum time one has to collect a debt. Consult the table below to check this law.

State	Oral Agreements	Written Contracts	Promissory Notes	Open Accounts
AL	6	6	6	3
AK	6	6	6	6
AZ	3	6	5	3
AR	3	5	6	3
CA	2	4	4	4
CO	6	6	6	6
CT	3	6	6	6

*Reported in years

(Continued text on following page)

State	Oral Agreements	Written Contracts	Promissory Notes	Open Accounts
DE	3	3	6	3
D.C.	3	3	3	3
FL	4	5	5	4
GA	4	6	6	4
HI	6	6	6	6
ID	4	5	10	4
IL	5	10	6	5
IN	6	10	10	6
IA	5	10	5	5
KS	3	5	5	3
KY	5	15	15	5
LA	10	10	10	3
ME	6	6	6	6
MD	3	3	6	3
MA	6	6	6	6
MI	6	6	6	6
MN	6	6	6	6
MS	3	3	3	3
MO	5	10	10	5
MT	5	8	8	5
NE	4	5	6	4
NV	4	6	3	4
NH	3	3	6	3
NJ	6	6	6	6
NM	4	6	6	4
NY	6	6	6	6
NC	3	3	5	3
ND	6	6	6	6

State	Oral Agreements	Written Contracts	Promissory Notes	Open Accounts
OH	6	15	15	—
OK	3	5	5	3
OR	6	6	6	6
PA	4	6	4	6
RI	15	15	10	10
SC	10	10	3	3
SD	6	6	6	6
TN	6	6	6	6
TX	4	4	4	4
UT	4	6	6	4
VT	6	6	5	6
VA	3	5	6	3
WA	3	6	6	3
WV	5	10	6	5
WI	6	6	10	6
WY	8	10	10	8

Collection Abbreviations

Abbreviation	Description
Atty	Place with attorney
B	Bankrupt
Bal	Balance
BTTR	Best time to reach
C	Collections
CB	Call back
CLM	Claim
DFB	Demand for balance

(Continued text on following page)

Abbreviation	Description
DC	Disconnected
EOM	End of month
EOW	End of week
FN	Final notice
HSB	Husband
HHC	Have husband call
HU	Hung up
INS	Insurance
IP	Insurance pending
L1, L2, L3	Letter 1, letter 2, letter 3
LB	Line busy
LM	Left message
LMVM	Left message, voice mail
MR	Mail return
NA	No answer
NFA	No forwarding address
NP	No phone
NSF	Nonsufficient funds
PA	Payment arrangement
PH	Phones
PF	Payment in full
PM	Payment in mail
PMT	Payment
PN	Private number
POE	Place of employment
POW	Payment on the way
PP	Partial payment
PT	Patient
S	Spouse

Abbreviation	Description
SEP	Separated
SK	Skipped town
TW	Talked with
UE	Unemployed
UTC	Unable to contact
VE	Verified employment
VI	Verified insurance

Bankruptcy

The types of bankruptcy are:

Type	Description
Chapter 7	All nonexempt assets of the patient are sold, with the proceeds distributed to the creditors. Secured creditors are first to be paid. Unsecured (like medical bills) are last to be paid. Chapter 7 is considered an absolute bankruptcy, in which many or all debts are wiped out.
Chapter 9	Not relevant for medical bills. Used for reorganization of a town.
Chapter 11	Not relevant for medical bills. Used for reorganization of a business, when it wants to continue doing business.
Chapter 12	Used for reorganization for a farmer who cannot meet financial obligations.
Chapter 13	Referred to as a "wage earner's bankruptcy." Protects the wage earner from creditors while the wage earner makes arrangements to repay all or some of the debts over 3–5 years. At the end of that time, the balance of what is owed on most debts is erased. Portion the bills (about 75%) over a fixed period.

Overpayments

An overpayment can result when:

■ Payment results from two different sources for the same service or procedure
■ Payment should have been sent to the patient
■ Payment resulted in more dollars than the allowed amount
■ Payment is the result of a computer or data entry error

All overpayments must be returned to the carrier within a reasonable amount of time (2–4 weeks). If a check is for multiple patients, make a copy of the check, and then deposit it. If a check is for one patient only, copy the check, and return it to the carrier. Attach a copy of the EOB/remittance advice so that the carrier can identify the patient. Keep a copy of all correspondence regarding this overpayment in a file.

Billing for Relatives

Medicare does not permit providers to bill for relatives or members of their households.

Household members would include anyone living in the house as part of the family, such as a nanny, maid, butler, chauffer, medical caregiver, or assistant. Individuals considered to be boarders (e.g., college students renting a room) would not be included. Relatives that are considered immediate are:

■ Spouse
■ Parent, child, brother, sister
■ Grandparents/grandchild and spouse
■ Stepparent, stepchild, stepbrother, stepsister

CPT (HCPCS Level I)

The CPT book is released in the later part of August or early September of each year. The codes in this book become effective on January 1 the following year. It is imperative that a new book be purchased each year due to revisions, new codes, and deleted codes.

Sections of the CPT Book

Code Range	Section Heading
99201–99499	Evaluation and Management
00100–01999 99100–99140	Anesthesiology
10021–69990	Surgery
70010–79999	Radiology
80048–89356	Laboratory/Pathology
90281–99199 99500–99602	Medicine

Each section contains guidelines for the codes in that specific section. These guidelines should be reviewed before using the codes.

In the event that a specific CPT code does not exist for the procedure performed, each section contains unlisted codes for this purpose. For example, unlisted procedure: pharynx, adenoids, or tonsils, 42999.

CPT Symbols

Symbol	Description
●	New code
▲	Revised code
▶ ◀	New or revised description
⊙	Codes include conscious sedation
⊘	Codes exempt from use of modifier -51
+	Codes that can be added onto a procedure or service

Clean Claim

A clean claim is one that has been submitted within the proper time and contains all the necessary information. This allows for the claim to be paid promptly, as additional information does not have to be requested. A clean claim means:

- It has no deficiencies and passes all the edits.
- The third-party carrier does not have to obtain additional information before processing the claim.
- The claim may be investigated in a "postpayment" state rather than payment being held until any investigation that may take place is completed.

Other claim-related terms:

- **Incomplete:** A claim that is missing required information; the provider is notified so that information can be sent
- **Rejected:** A claim that requires investigation and needs further clarification; this claim must be resubmitted with the necessary information
- **Invalid:** A claim that contains complete, necessary information but is still incorrect; this claim must be resubmitted with the proper corrections
- **Dirty:** A claim submitted with errors; a claim that requires manual processing; or a claim that has been rejected for payment
- **Dingy:** A claim that cannot be processed for the service or procedure or bill type
- **Paper:** A claim that is submitted on paper, whether typed or computer-generated
- **Electronic:** A claim that is submitted to the carrier through a central processing unit or via telephone line or direct wire

Locum Tenens Providers

Locum tenens providers cover a physician during periods of illness, pregnancy, or vacation. The locum tenens covers the physician's practice and treat patients as if the practice was their own. Established patients are still billed as established patients, as all billing is reported under the regular physician. See the following listing of conditions that must be met to bill for locum tenens:

- The patient's regular physician is not available.
- The regular physician pays the locum tenens a per diem fee.
- The locum tenens cannot provide services to Medicare patients for more than 60 days.
- Services by the locum tenens are billed using modifier -Q6 in Box 24d of the CMS 1500 form.

Managed Care

Summary of Managed Care Plans

Summary of most common types of managed care plans:

- HMO-health maintenance organization
- PPO-preferred provider organization
- IPA-independent practice association
- EPO-exclusive provider organization
- POS-point of service

Managed Care Plan	Co-pay Deductible	Payment	Authorization Required
HMO	Co-pay is fixed	Capitated Fee for service carve-outs	Yes
PPO	Co-pay is fixed Deductible	Fee for service	Yes
IPA	Co-pay is fixed	Capitated Fee for service carve-outs	Yes
EPO	Co-pay is fixed	Capitated Fee for service carve-outs	Yes
POS	Co-pay is fixed Deductible	Capitated Fee for service carve-outs	Yes

Do's and Don'ts of Working with Managed Care

Do:

- Label each patient's chart with the name of the patient's managed care organization.
- Bill each organization the same day of the service.
- Monitor the number of days it takes to be paid under a fee-for-service method. Document any late capitation checks. Promptly call your provider representative with the results.
- Appeal inconsistent fee-for-service payments for the CPT code or unreasonable payments inconsistent with the contracted fee schedule.
- Appeal problem payment decisions directly to the medical director of each organization.
- Request financial reports each year and have the doctors review them before contacting time.
- Network with other practices involved with the problem managed care organization.
- Read the regulations and requirements of the managed care carrier and incorporate them into the policy and procedure manual of the practice.

Don't:

- Bill a patient who is a member of a managed care organization unless it is for a deductible, co-payment, or excluded benefit.
- Let your doctors accept the decision of a nurse reviewer if you believe the patient's care would be compromised. Have your doctor always speak to a medical director when services have been denied.
- Let the doctors discharge a patient or cancel a test they believe is medically necessary when benefits have been denied.
- Discuss the managed care carrier negatively with your patients.
- Discriminate against managed care organization patients by not giving them timely appointments.

Quick Guide to Managed Care

Entity	Advantages	Disadvantages
Patient	Cost reduction Better benefits	Less attention Restricted use of providers General confusion
Managed care plan	Fixed rates Cost reduction Easy claim payment Small number of providers	Contract demands Adverse member reactions Multiple contract rates
Hospital	Possible volume increase Prompt payment	Reduced fees Contract demands Complex billing
Physician	Possible volume increase Prompt payment Maintaining current patients	Reduced fees Contract demands Complex billing Upsets patient relations Upsets referral patterns

Medicare

Nonparticipating Providers

Providers that do not participate in Medicare are subject to a certain dollar amount that they can charge. This charge is referred to as a "limiting charge." The Medicare Fee Schedule contains a column listing the limiting charge. A Federal law prohibits a nonparticipating provider from charging more than this limiting charge.

Deductibles and Co-pays

Medicare deductibles and co-pays cannot be waived on a routine basis. If this should occur, the practice could be in violation of the Anti-Kickback Statute or False Claims Act.

(Continued text on following page)

The listing below contains examples of inappropriate waiving of Medicare deductibles and co-pays.

- Routine reason of "financial hardship" given to patients without proper investigation of finances
- Routine waiving of a specific group of individuals in order to obtain additional patients (for example, all Medicare patients living in a particular senior home)

Medicare Secondary Payor (MSP)

There are cases where another health insurance pays before the patient's Medicare benefits. In these cases, the other health insurance is primary, with Medicare being the secondary insurance. This situation occurs under the following conditions:

MSP Billing Guide	
Primary Insurer: Medicare	**Primary Insurer: Other Insurance**
The patient is 65 years or older and is retired or disabled.	The patient is 65 years or older and is still employed and covered under an employer's insurance contract.
The patient works for the military and carries Tricare insurance coverage. Medicare is primary, and Tricare is secondary.	The patient has Veterans Administration benefits that cover all services and procedures.
The patient has Medicaid. Medicaid becomes the secondary payor and covers patient's deductible.	The patient has Railroad Retirement benefits.
The patient is 65 years or older and retired. The patient's spouse works but has no health insurance coverage through the employer.	The patient is 65 years or older and retired. The patient's spouse works and both the spouse and patient have coverage through the spouse's employer.

Primary Insurer: Medicare	Primary Insurance: Other Insurance
The patient has coverage under a self-employed plan, such as real estate agents.	■ The patient is a member of the United Mine Workers of America. ■ The patient's injury or condition is a result of a motor vehicle accident. ■ The patient's injury or condition is a result of employment.

Physician Assistant (PA) Billing

Medicare pays the PAs' employers in all settings at 85% of the physician's fee schedule. This includes:

- Hospitals (inpatient, outpatient, and emergency departments)
- Nursing facilities
- Home
- Offices and clinics
- First assisting at surgery

Important billing facts:

- Assignment is mandatory; state law determines supervision and scope of practice
- Medicare pays the PAs' employers for medical services provided

Setting	Supervision Requirement	Reimbursement Rate	Services
Office/clinic when physician is not on site	State law	85% of physician's fee schedule	All the services the PA is legally authorized to provide that would have been covered if provided personally by a physician
Office/clinic when physician is on site	Physician must be in the suite of the office	100% of physician's fee schedule	Same as above
Home visit House call	State law	85% of physician's fee schedule	Same as above
Skilled nursing facility and nursing facility	State law	85% of physician's fee schedule	Same as above
Hospital	State law	85% of physician's fee schedule	Same as above
First assisting at surgery in all settings	State law	85% of physician's first assistant fee schedule	Same as above
Federally certified rural health clinics	State law	Cost-based reimbursement	Same as above
HMO	State law	Reimbursement is on capitation basis	All services contracted for as part of an HMO contract

Nurse Practitioner (NP) Billing

Important Facts:

- NPs must submit their own billing number for all professional services "furnished in facility or other provider settings."
- A UPIN billing number must be obtained and submitted on all claims. In situations when NPs are members of a group practice, enter the group practice PIN number on one line of the claim form and the NP UPIN on another.
- Modifiers are now applicable only when submitting "assistant at surgery" claims.
- Payments to NPs now equal "80 percent of the lesser of either the actual charge or 85 percent of the physician fee schedule amount.
- For assistant at surgery services, payments equal 80 percent of the lesser of either the actual charge or 85 percent of the physician fee schedule amount paid to a physician serving as an assistant at surgery."
- NPs will be unable, however, to receive separate Medicare payments in rural health clinic (RHC) and federally qualified health center (FQHC) settings.

Medicare Fee Schedule

There are three reimbursement columns in a Medicare fee schedule:

PAR	Participating provider fee
Non-PAR	Nonparticipating provider fee
LC	Limiting charge fee

Medical Supplies and Equipment

Medicare can be billed for any supply and equipment that will be used in a patient's home. Medicare's definition of a home includes the following locations:

(Continued text on following page)

- The patient's home
- A relative's home where the patient is living
- A home for senior citizens
- A homeless shelter

Nursing homes cannot be considered a patient's home and therefore medical supplies and equipment cannot be billed.

Medicare Covered/Noncovered Services

Some of the most common covered and noncovered services are listed in the following table. The Medicare manual for each state provides a comprehensive listing of these services.

Medicare Part B Covered Services	Medicare Part B Noncovered Services
Provider services (office visits, hospital visits, consultations, nursing home visits, etc.)	Cosmetic surgery
X-rays, laboratory testing, PT, OT, and other outpatient diagnostic testing	Dental services
Ambulatory surgical center (ASC) services	Custodial care
Surgical dressings, casts, splints, etc.	Services resulting from workers compensation or motor vehicle accident
Certain braces	Services deemed not medically necessary
Durable medical equipment	Routine physical examinations

Medicare Billing Summary

CMS-1500 form is used to submit claims	Deductibles: $100 for physician services and out-patients	Allowable fees will vary according to the plan. Most use Usual, Customary, and Reasonable basis	A Surgical Financial Disclosure Form is required for all nonassigned claims of $500 or more
Deadline for processing claims is Dec. 31 of the year following the DOS	A minimum of 45 days must pass before a claim can be submitted	Coalminer claims sent to: Federal Black Lung Program Box 828 Lanham-Seabrook, MD 20703-0828	Durable medical equipment (DME) claims must be sent to the appropriate DME regional carrier

Medicare Review Process

The following steps illustrate the Medicare review process. The Medicare Manual in each state provides the details necessary to begin this process.

Steps	Action	Key Points
1	Review	■ Claim must be requested within 6 months of the date on the Explanation of Benefits.
2	Fair hearing	■ Claim must be requested in writing within 6 months of the result of the review. ■ Claim must exceed $100 in amount. ■ Hearings take place over the phone, face to face, or on the record (where the decision is automatically based on the facts submitted).

(Continued text on following page)

Steps	Action	Key Points
3	Administrative law judge hearing	■ Claim must be requested in writing within 60 days of the result of the fair hearing. ■ Claim must exceed $500 in amount.
4	Appeals council review	■ Claim must be requested in writing through the Social Security Administration (SSA) Office of Hearings and Appeals within 60 days of the result of the administrative law judge hearing. ■ Claim must exceed $500 in amount.
5	Federal district court hearing	■ Civil action must be filed in federal district court within 60 days of the result of the Appeals Council decision. ■ The claimant must be represented by an attorney.

Advance Beneficiary Notice (ABN)

When a service is provided to a Medicare patient that Medicare considers not medically necessary, the physician should notify the patient by using an Advance Beneficiary Notice (ABN). This notice must be completed, signed, and dated. The modifier -GA must be used when submitting the claim for a service or procedure where an ABN is on file in the physician's office. The following list contains a list of reasons that the physician practice believes the service or procedure may not be covered. This reason must be stated clearly on the ABN that the patient signs.

1. Medicare does not usually pay for this many services
2. Medicare does not usually pay for this service
3. Medicare does not pay for this because it is a treatment that has not been proven effective
4. Medicare does not pay for such extensive treatment(s)
5. Medicare does not pay for this equipment for the diagnosis stated
6. Medicare does not pay for this many services within the period reported

These ABN notices should be completed by all Medicare patients, only when there is a possibility of noncoverage of the service or procedure. Having patients sign ABNs blanketly is not a good practice.

Medicaid

Medicaid Services Available

- Inpatient and outpatient services
- Physician visits
- Dental visits (surgical)
- Nursing facility services for those over age 21 years
- Home health for those eligible for a skilled nursing facility
- Family planning and supplies
- Rural health clinics
- Laboratory tests and x-rays
- NP services
- Federally qualified health center
- Nurse midwife services
- Early and periodic screening, diagnosis, and treatment (EPSDT) services for individuals under age 21 years.

Confirming Medicaid Eligibility	
Steps	**Procedure**
Step 1	The patient must present a valid ID card.
Step 2	Eligibility can change monthly as it is based on monthly income, so always verify using the dedicated phone line.
Step 3	Confirmation of eligibility should be obtained and maintained in the patient's chart in case of future denial of claim.
Step 4	Confirmation can also be obtained through a "swipe" box. A print-out will indicate coverage.
Step 5	Retroactive eligibility is sometimes granted to patients whose income has fallen below the "state-set" eligibility level and who had high medical expenses prior to filing for Medicaid.
Step 6	The office must verify any patient notification of retroactive eligibility. If the patient made payments for services during that time, the payments must be returned to the patient, and Medicaid should be billed.

Preauthorization

Some states have placed their Medicaid plans into an HMO. These HMOs require preauthorization services, which include:

- Elective admissions
  - Reason for inpatient treatment
  - Admission diagnosis and outline of treatment plan
- Emergency admissions
  - Medical justification for inpatient treatment
  - Date of admission
- Admission diagnosis and outline of treatment plan

- Preoperation days more than 1
  - Reason why surgery cannot be performed within 24 hours of time when need was established
  - Number of additional days requested
- Outpatient procedure performed as inpatient procedure
  - Code and description of surgical procedure
  - Medical justification for performing the surgery on an inpatient basis
  - Exceeding hospital stay limit (set by state) due to complications
- Beginning and ending dates originally authorized
- Statement describing the complications
- Date complications presented
- Diagnosis for first illness
- Diagnosis stated on original preauthorization request
- Diagnosis for secondary disorder

Extension of Inpatient Days
- Medical necessity for the extension
- Number of additional days requested
- Basis for approval of more than 1 preoperation day
- Performance of multiple procedures that, when combined, necessitate a length of stay in excess of that required for any one individual procedure

Development of postoperative complications or a medical history that dictates longer than usual postoperative observation by medical staff

---

NB Billing Center

Important facts:

- 50 states cover medical services provided by PAs under their Medicaid programs.
- The rate of reimbursement, which is paid to the employing practice and not directly to the PA, is either the same as or slightly lower than that paid to physicians.

NP Billing

Important facts:

- Federal law mandates direct reimbursement to pediatric (PNP) and family (FNP) nurse practitioners providing services to children.
- Physician collaboration is not required within the federal mandate.
- Each state determines the reimbursement rate for NPs.

Medicaid Billing Summary

CMS-1500 form is used to submit claims	Deadlines for processing claims is determined by each state	All nonemergency hospitalizations must be preauthorized	Allowable fees vary according to each state
A minimum of 45 days must pass before a claim can be resubmitted	Deductibles: there is a deductible for patients who are medically indigent.	Co-payments are required by most states, generally ranging $2–$10 per encounter	There is no Medicaid premium

Tricare

TRICARE is a health-care program for:

- Active duty members of the military and qualified family members
- CHAMPUS-eligible retirees and qualified family members
- Eligible survivors of members of the uniformed services

It consists of three plans with varying benefits:

1. TRICARE Prime
2. TRICARE Extra
3. TRICARE Standard

TRICARE differs from other insurance carriers as the **fiscal year for collecting deductibles runs from October 1 through September 30.**

PA Billing

Important facts:

- TRICARE covers all medically necessary services provided by a PA.
- The PA must be supervised in accordance with state law.
- The supervising physician must be an authorized TRICARE provider.
- **The employer bills for the services provided by the PA.**
- The allowable charge for all medical services provided by PAs under TRICARE Standard, the fee-for service program, except assisting at surgery, is 85% of the allowable fee for comparable services rendered by a physician in a similar location.
- Reimbursement for assisting at surgery is 65% of the physician's allowable fee for comparable services.
- PAs are eligible providers of care under TRICARE's two managed care programs, TRICARE Prime and Extra.
  - TRICARE Prime is similar to an HMO.
  - TRICARE Extra is run like a preferred provider organization in which practitioners agree to accept a predetermined discounted fee for their services.

Workers Compensation

Eligibility consists of an on-the-job injury or a condition that is the direct result of the individual's job.

The law states that a waiting period must elapse before income benefits are payable. This period is determined by each individual state.

(Continued text on following page)

Classifications of workers compensation consist of:

- Medical claims with no disability
- Temporary disability
- Permanent disability
- Vocational rehabilitation
- Death of a worker

The provider must accept workers compensation as payment in full and cannot bill any additional fees.

Fees are reimbursed either by the Medicare fee schedule or by a private fee schedule and are determined by each individual state.

Miscellaneous Terms/Facts

- **Guarantor:** the individual who is responsible for payment of the medical bill. For children to be guarantors, they must be either 18 or 21 years of age (depending on the state regulations)
- **Major Medical:** an insurance policy that covers medical expenses resulting from catastrophic or prolonged illness/injuries or coverage for such things as office visits that are not included in the plan's coverage

Miscellaneous Facts

- Claims denied as "not medically necessary" cannot be billed to the patient unless an advance beneficiary notice has been completed acknowledging the patient's understanding of the service and why it may or may not be covered. The burden of medical necessity is placed on the provider and is the primary reason for Medicare denials across the country.
- Use an Evaluation and Management (E&M) code when pronouncing death of a patient.

Evaluation and Management Services

Evaluation and Management (E&M) codes are Current Procedural Terminology (CPT) codes (Current Procedural Terminology, ©2005 American Medical Association, All Rights Reserved), used for the reporting of certain services such as office visits, consultations, inpatient services, emergency room services, nursing facility services, domiciliary care services, and home services. Each category of E&M service contains two to seven levels for billing. Each level requires a specific amount of documentation to be billable.

These services are listed below in the Table of Evaluation and Management Services.

CPT Codes	Description
99201–99205	New patient office visit codes
99211–99215	Established patient office visit codes
99221–99223	Initial hospital service
99231–99233	Subsequent hospital service
99241–99245	Consultation, outpatient
99251–99255	Consultation, inpatient
99261–99263	Consultation, follow-up hospital
99271–99275	Consultation, confirmatory
99234–99236	Hospital Observation or inpatient care services
99217–99220	Hospital Observation services
99281–99285	Emergency room services
99301–99303	Initial comprehensive nursing facility service
99311–99313	Subsequent nursing facility service
99341–99345	Home services, new patient
99347–99350	Home services, established patient
99321–99323	New patient
99331–99333	Established patient

(Continued text on following page)

CPT Codes	Description
99381–99387	Preventive med codes, new patient
99391–99397	Preventive med codes, established patient
99354–99355	Prolonged care, outpatient
99356–99357	Prolonged care, inpatient
99358–99359	Prolonged care, without direct patient contact

*Current Procedural Terminology © 2006 American Medical Association,
All Rights Reserved.

The Principles of Documentation were released in 1995 as
collaboration between the American Medical Association (AMA)
and the Centers for Medicare & Medicaid Services (CMS, known
then as the Health Care Finance Administration). These
guidelines were revised in 1997 and 2000 and are still
undergoing revisions. Until the final guidelines are released,
CMS instructs providers to use either the 1995 or 1997
guidelines; the decision is the provider's.

Principles of Documentation

The medical record:
1. is a tool of clinical care and communication.
2. should be complete and legible.
3. should include as documentation:
   a. reason for the visit; appropriate history, physical
      examination, review of diagnostic test results, and any
      other ancillary services.
   b. provider's assessment of the patient's condition, clinical
      impressions or diagnoses.
   c. plan of care/treatment plan.
   d. date and legible identity of the person who provided the
      service.
4. should contain the rationale for ordering diagnostic services.
5. should contain accessibility to past and present diagnoses.
6. should contain appropriate health risk factors.
7. should contain the patient's progress, responses to treatment,
   and complications and changes in treatment or diagnoses.

8. should support the CPT and ICD-9 codes billed.
9. should be confidential.

Components of E&M Services

1. History
2. Examination
3. Medical Decision Making
4. Counseling
5. Coordination of Care
6. Nature of Presenting Problem
7. Time

In the table above, the first three components are key components (history, examination, and medical decision making) of E&M services and are required in most categories of E&M codes.

Time

Time, which is No. 7 on the list, is a consideration only if counseling is 50% or more of the visit.

Some CPT codes are time-based codes. Time-based codes reflect the time associated with the service provided. Some time-based codes are used to report episodes of Critical Care, Prolonged care, and Psychology service areas.

The only time-based codes listed in the Table of Evaluation and Management Services are the prolonged care codes. When choosing an E&M code based on time, the documentation requirements are very specific. The documentation in the medical record must show that counseling is 50% or more of the visit. For example, a note should look like this:

"I spent 45 minutes with Barbara Smith and her husband today. Of that 45 minutes, 30 minutes were spent discussing the results of her abnormal echocardiogram."

The note should then provide a summary of the key components of the discussion. This documentation indicates that counseling was more than 50% of the visit.

The following note does not meet this criterion:

"I spent 30 minutes with Barbara discussing the results of her abnormal echocardiogram."

(Continued text on following page)

This note does not indicate that the time spent counseling Barbara Smith was 50% or greater than the total time of the office visit.

History

There are four **levels** of history:

1. Problem focused
2. Expanded problem focused
3. Detailed
4. Comprehensive

Within these four **levels**, there are four **elements** of history:

1. Chief complaint
2. History of present illness
3. Review of systems
4. Past, family, and social history

Chief Complaint (written as cc)

The chief complaint is the reason for the visit, or why the patient sought care. This is generally in the patient's own words and is a short phrase or two. It is important to be specific when documenting this element and not to use vague language as this may disqualify the patient encounter for reimbursement.

For example, the list below illustrates language that is vague; it does not state why the patient sought care.

Incorrect:

- cc - check-up
- Follow-up visit
- ✓ up
- Routine visit

Correct:

- cc - check-up on high blood pressure
- Follow-up visit for back pain
- ✓ up on diabetes
- Routine visit for reflux

History of Present Illness (written as HPI)

The HPI is a description of the present illness from the beginning of symptoms to the time of the patient encounter. There are eight elements of the HPI. They are:

1. Location
2. Quality
3. Severity
4. Duration
5. Timing
6. Context
7. Modifying factors
8. Associated signs and symptoms

There are two levels of HPI:

1. Brief: documentation of 1 to 3 elements from the list.
2. Extended: documentation of 4 or more elements from the list.

A brief history focuses on the patient's problem, whereas an extended history goes beyond that to obtain information that may support multiple diagnoses. An example of a brief HPI is as follows:

cc - complaining of knee pain
HPI - pain has been present in left knee
   (location) for 2 weeks (timing)

In the above example, left knee is the location and 2 weeks is the timing. Two elements of HPI are met: location and timing. Continuing to build on this note will provide more information about the patient's complaint and justify an extended HPI. See the following example:

cc - complaining of knee pain
HPI - pain has been present in left knee (location) for 2 weeks (timing). Pt states that pain has gotten so severe (severity) that Advil used to help but now doesn't (modifying factors). Pt reports pain started when she played softball (context) with her son and fell while running to a base.

(Continued text on following page)

In the above note, left knee is the location and 2 weeks is the timing; pain is so severe, Advil does not relieve it anymore; pain started when playing softball. In this note, five elements of HPI are met, location, timing, severity, modifying factors, and context.

Review of Systems (written as ROS)

An ROS is an accounting of signs and symptoms of various organ systems obtained through a series of questions. There are 14 systems contained in an ROS. These systems are:

The 14 Systems of ROS

1. Constitutional
2. Eyes
3. Ears/nose/mouth/throat
4. Cardiovascular
5. Respiratory
6. Gastrointestinal
7. Genitourinary
8. Musculoskeletal
9. Integumentary
10. Neurological
11. Psychiatric
12. Endocrine
13. Hematological/lymphatic
14. Allergic/immunological

The Three Levels of ROS

1. Problem pertinent: Review and documentation of one system
2. Extended: Review and documentation of two to nine systems
3. Complete: Review and documentation of at least 10 systems

A problem pertinent ROS involves a review of system(s) that can be affected by, play a role in, or is (are) likely to be involved in the patient's problem. An extended review includes a more in-depth review of system(s). A complete review includes 10 of the 14 systems listed above. This type of review is considered comprehensive in nature.

Past, Family, Social History (written as PFSH)

A past history contains information about the patient's past experiences with illnesses, injuries, and treatments. This may include information about the following:

- Hospitalizations
- Illnesses and/or injuries
- Surgeries
- Current medications
- Allergies to drugs or the environment
- Age-appropriate immunization status
- Age-appropriate dietary or feeding status

A family history contains information about the patient's family. This may include such information as:

- Diseases of the mother, father, siblings, and/or children
- Health status or cause of death of any of the above
- Diseases of family members that may be hereditary or cause the patient to be at risk

A social history contains information about past or current activities and/or conditions. This may include such information as:

- Marital status
- Employment
- Use of controlled substances
- Use of alcohol
- Living arrangements
- Current employment
- Occupational history
- Level of education
- Sexual history

The Two Levels of PFSH

1. Pertinent: Documentation of one history area
2. Complete: Documentation of two to three history areas

A complete history must contain the documentation of either two or three history areas, depending on the category of E&M service. The following tables identify which type of service requires the documentation of three history areas (3 out of 3 rule) and which types of service require the documentation of two history areas (2 out of 3 rule).

(Continued text on following page)

3 out of 3 Rule
When the service type is one of an "initial" contact, all three history areas must be documented.

Visit Types

1. New office service
2. Consultation, outpatient
3. Consultation, inpatient
4. Consultation, confirmatory
5. Initial hospital service
6. Initial nursing facility service
7. Home services, new patient
8. Observation services
9. Observation services or inpatient hospital

2 out of 3 Rule
When the service type is one of an established service, only two of the three history areas must be documented.

Visit Types

1. Established office service
2. Consultation, follow-up inpatient
3. Subsequent hospital service
4. Subsequent nursing facility service
5. Home services, established patient
6. Emergency room services

History Summary				
Type of History	**CC**	**HPI**	**ROS**	**PFSH**
Problem focused	Present	Brief	N/A	N/A
Expanded problem focused	Present	Brief	Problem pertinent	N/A
Detailed	Present	Extended	Extended	Pertinent
Comprehensive	Present	Extended	Complete	Comprehensive

Examination

The examination portion of the visit contains documentation of the objective findings of the provider of the service. There are currently two sets of examination guidelines: those of 1995 and 1997. The 1995 guidelines are somewhat subjective, whereas the 1997 guidelines are very specific. The provider of the service may choose which guideline set he/she wants to use.

1995 Examination Guidelines

Level	Description
Problem focused	A limited examination of the affected body area or organ system
Expanded problem focused	A limited examination of the affected body area or organ system and other symptomatic or related organ systems
Detailed	An extended examination of the affected body area(s) and other symptomatic or related organ system(s)
Comprehensive	A general multisystem examination or a complete examination of a single organ system

Body areas:
- Chest
- Abdomen
- Back (including spine)
- Neck
- Genitalia, groin, buttocks
- Head (including face)
- Extremities; each one is an area

Organ Systems:
- Constitutional
- Eyes
- Ears/Nose/Mouth/Throat
- Cardiovascular
- Respiratory
- Gastrointestinal
- Genitourinary
- Musculoskeletal
- Integumentary
- Neurological
- Psychiatric
- Hematological/lymphatic/immunological

1997 Examination Guidelines

The 1997 examination guidelines contain a multisystem examination, plus 10 single specialty examinations. These examinations are as follows:

General Multisystem

1. Cardiovascular
2. Ears/Nose/Mouth/Throat
3. Eye
4. Genitourinary
5. Hematological/Lymphatic/Immunologic
6. Musculoskeletal
7. Neurological
8. Psychiatric
9. Respiratory
10. Integumentary

Under the general multisystem examination, the following requirements must be met:

Level	Description
Problem focused	Perform and document 1 to 5 elements identified by a bullet.
Expanded problem focused	Perform and document at least 6 elements identified by a bullet.
Detailed	Perform and document at least 2 elements identified by a bullet from each of 6 areas/systems or at least 12 elements identified by a bullet in 2 or more areas/systems.
Comprehensive	Perform all elements identified by a bullet in at least 9 organ systems or body areas and document at least 2 elements identified by a bullet from each of 9 areas/systems.

A detailed listing of these requirements by body areas and organ systems can be found in the Federal Register.

Under the specialty guidelines, the following requirements must be met:

Level	Description
Problem focused	Perform and document 1 to 5 elements identified by a bullet.
Expanded problem focused	Perform and document at least 6 elements identified by a bullet.
Detailed	Perform and document at least 12 elements identified by a bullet.
Comprehensive	Perform all elements identified by a bullet and document every italicized element in a shaded area and at least 1 nonitalicized element in each of the nonshaded areas.

Medical Decision Making

The medical decision making portion of the visit entails the complexity of establishing the diagnosis and/or management option(s). Medical decision making is measured by the following:

- The number of diagnoses and/or management options
- The amount and/or complexity of medical records, diagnostic tests, and other information to be reviewed and analyzed
- The risk of significant complications and morbidity and/or mortality rates

The Four Levels of Medical Decision Making

Level	Number of Diagnoses/ Management Options	Amount and/ or Complexity of Data Reviewed	Risk of Complication and/or Morbidity or Mortality Rate
Straight-forward	Minimal	Minimal/None	Minimal
Low complexity	Limited	Limited/Low	Low
Moderate complexity	Multiple	Moderate	Moderate
High complexity	Extensive	Extensive	High

(Continued text on following page)

MGMT SURG

Two of the three indicators will establish the level of medical decision making.

If a patient presents with multiple diagnoses and multiple management options must be considered, the complexity of the medical decision making is increased. The amount and/or complexity of data that must be obtained, reviewed, and analyzed during the patient encounter must be clear and concise. For test results, document thought processes, analysis, and evaluation of both positive and negative findings. Their impact on treatment should be documented. Review of the patient medical record, past and present, should be documented with comments. Note the extent of records and data that are reviewed with an analysis. The potential risk to the patient is an important element in assessing the complexity of this key component of medical decision making. The following table can be used to identify risk:

Type of Problem	Description
Minimal	May not require presence of physician, but service provided under physician's supervision
Self-limited/ minor	Runs definite and prescribed course; transient in nature and not likely to permanently alter health status; or has a good prognosis with management/compliance
Low severity	Low risk of morbidity without treatment; little to no risk of mortality without treatment; full recovery without functional impairment expected
Moderate severity	Moderate risk of morbidity without treatment; moderate risk of mortality without treatment; uncertain prognosis or increased probability of prolonged functional impairment
High severity	High to extreme risk of morbidity; moderate to high risk of mortality without treatment or high probability of severe, prolonged functional impairment

Examples of various types of risk are illustrated below

Level of Risk	Presenting Problems	Diagnostic Procedures Ordered	Management Options Selected
Minimal	Insect bite, cold, tinea corporis	ECG, chest x-ray, KOH, UA	Rest, gargle, bandages
Low	Cystitis, sprains, controlled DM, controlled BP	Pulmonary functions, BE, skin biopsies	OTC drugs, PT, OT, IV fluids, minor surgery/ no risk
Moderate	Lump in breast, colitis, pneumonia	Arteriogram, lumbar puncture, endoscopies/no risk	Rx management, IV fluids w/ medications, closed treatment of fracture, elective major surgery
High	Acute MI, psychiatric illness w/ threat, TIA, trauma	CV imaging studies w/ contrast, endoscopies w/risk	Emergency major surgeries, DNRs, monitoring toxic drugs

Medical Necessity

Although the service may contain a properly documented history, examination, and medical decision making, if there is no medical necessity for the level of service chosen for billing, the service may be downcoded by the carrier. The government's definition of medical necessity is a service that is reasonable and necessary for the diagnosis or treatment of illness or injury or to improve the functioning of a malformed body member.

			The Decision Matrix for New Office Patients			
Code	History	Exam	Medical Decision Making	Nature of Presenting Problem	Counseling/ Coordination of Care	Time
99201	Problem focused	Problem focused	Straightforward	Self-limited/ minor	Yes	10
99202	Expanded problem focused	Expanded problem focused	Straightforward	Low to moderate	Yes	20
99203	Detailed	Detailed	Low	Moderate	Yes	30
99204	Compre-hensive	Compre-hensive	Moderate	Moderate to high	Yes	45
99205	Compre-hensive	Compre-hensive	High	High	Yes	60

Requires all three key components to be documented

			Medical Decision Making	Nature of Presenting Problem	Counseling/ Coordination of Care	Time
Code	History	Exam				
99211	Generally does not require a physician			Minimal	No	5
99212	Problem focused	Problem focused	Straightforward	Self-limited/ minor	Yes	10
99213	Expanded problem focused	Expanded problem focused	Low	Low to moderate	Yes	15
99214	Detailed	Detailed	Moderate	Moderate to high	Yes	25
99215	Comprehensive	Comprehensive	High	Moderate to high	Yes	40

The Decision Matrix for Established Office Patients

Requires all two of the three key components to be documented

The Decision Matrix for Initial Hospital Patients						
Code	History	Exam	Medical Decision Making	Nature of Presenting Problem	Counseling/ Coordination of Care	Time
99221	Detailed/ Compre-hensive	Detailed/ Compre-hensive	Straightforward or low	Low	Yes	30
99222	Compre-hensive	Compre-hensive	Moderate	Moderate	Yes	50
99223	Compre-hensive	Compre-hensive	High	High	Yes	70

Requires all three key components to be documented

MGMT SURG

			Medical Decision Making	Nature of Presenting Problem	Counseling/ Coordination of Care	Time
Code	History	Exam				
99231	Problem focused	Problem focused	Straightfor-ward/Low	Patient is stable, recover-ing, or improving	Yes	15
99232	Expanded problem focused	Expanded problem focused	Moderate	Responding inadequately or minor complication	Yes	25
99233	Detailed	Detailed	High	Unstable or developed significant complication of problem	Yes	35

The Decision Matrix for Subsequent Hospital Patients

Requires two of the three key components to be documented

The Decision Matrix for Consultation, Outpatient

Code	History	Exam	Medical Decision Making	Nature of Presenting Problem	Counseling/ Coordination of Care	Time
99241	Problem focused	Problem focused	Straightforward	Self-limited/ minor	Yes	15
99242	Expanded problem focused	Expanded problem focused	Straightforward	Low	Yes	30
99243	Detailed	Detailed	Low	Moderate	Yes	40
99244	Comprehensive	Comprehensive	Moderate	Moderate to high	Yes	60
99245	Comprehensive	Comprehensive	High	Moderate to high	Yes	80

Requires all three key components to be documented

		The Decision Matrix for Consultation, Inpatient				
Code	History	Exam	Medical Decision Making	Nature of Presenting Problem	Counseling/ Coordination of Care	Time
99251	Problem focused	Problem focused	Straightforward	Self-limited/ minor	Yes	20
99252	Expanded problem focused	Expanded problem focused	Straightforward	Low	Yes	40
99253	Detailed	Detailed	Low	Moderate	Yes	55
99254	Compre-hensive	Compre-hensive	Moderate	Moderate to high	Yes	80
99255	Compre-hensive	Compre-hensive	High	Moderate to high	Yes	110

Requires all three key components to be documented

Code	History	Examination	Medical Decision Making	Nature of Presenting Problem	Counseling/ Coordination of Care	Time
The Decision Matrix for Consultation, Follow-Up Inpatient						
99261	Problem focused	Problem focused	Straightfor- ward/Low	Patient is stable, recovering, or improving	Consistent with nature of problems	10
99262	Expanded problem focused	Expanded problem focused	Moderate	Responding inadequately or developed minor com- plication	Consistent with nature of problems	20
99263	Detailed	Detailed	High	Unstable or developed significant complication or new signifi- cant problem	Consistent with nature of problems	30

Requires two of the three key components to be documented

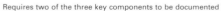

The Decision Matrix for Consultation, Confirmatory

Code	History	Exam	Medical	Nature of Presenting Problem	Counseling/ Coordination of Care
99271	Problem focused	Problem focused	Straightforward	Self-limited/ minor	Yes
99272	Expanded problem focused	Expanded problem focused	Straightforward	Low	Yes
99273	Detailed	Detailed	Low	Moderate	Yes
99274	Comprehensive	Comprehensive	Moderate	Moderate to high	Yes
99275	Comprehensive	Comprehensive	High	Moderate to high	Yes

Requires all three key components to be documented

MGMT SURG

		The Decision Matrix for Hospital Observation or Inpatient Care			
Code	History	Exam	Medical Decision Making	Nature of Presenting Problem	Counseling/ Coordination of Care
99234	Detailed/Comprehensive	Detailed/Comprehensive	Straightforward or low	Low	Consistent with nature of problems
99235	Comprehensive	Comprehensive	Moderate	Moderate	Consistent with nature of problems
99236	Comprehensive	Comprehensive	High	High	Consistent with nature of problems

Requires all three key components to be documented

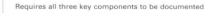

			Medical Decision Making	Nature of Presenting Problem	Counseling/ Coordination of Care
Code	History	Exam			
The Decision Matrix for Hospital Observation or Inpatient Care					
99218	Detailed/Com-prehensive	Detailed/Comp-rehensive	Straightforward or Low	Low	Consistent with nature of problems
99219	Comprehensive	Comprehensive	Moderate	Moderate	Consistent with nature of problems
99220	Comprehensive	Comprehensive	High	High	Consistent with nature of problems
99217	Discharge Day: Can be used only if discharge is on other than the initial date of observation status				
Requires all three key components to be documented					

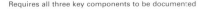

		The Decision Matrix for Emergency Room Services			
Code	History	Exam	Medical Decision Making	Nature of Presenting Problem	Counseling/ Coordination of Care
99281	Problem focused	Problem focused	Straightforward	Self-limited/ minor	Consistent with nature of problems
99282	Expanded problem focused	Expanded problem focused	Low	Low to Moderate	Consistent with nature of problems
99283	Expanded problem focused	Expanded problem focused	Moderate	Moderate	Consistent with nature of problems
99284	Detailed	Detailed	Moderate	High	Consistent with nature of problems
99285	Comprehensive	Comprehensive	High	High	Consistent with nature of problems
Requires two of the three key components to be documented					

The Decision Matrix for Initial Nursing Facility						
Comprehensive New or Established	History	Exam	Medical Decision Making	Nature of Presenting Problem	Counseling/ Coordination of Care	Time
99301	Detailed	Compre-hensive	Straightforward or low	Moderate to high	Yes	30
99302	Detailed	Compre-hensive	Moderate to high	Moderate to high	Yes	40
99303	Compre-hensive	Compre-hensive	Moderate to high	Moderate to high	Yes	50

Requires all three key components to be documented

MGMT SURG

MEMT SURG

The Decision Matrix for Subsequent Nursing Facility						
Subsequent New or Established	History	Exam	Medical Decision Making	Nature of Presenting Problem	Counseling/ Coordination of Care	Time
99311	Problem focused	Problem focused	Straight-forward	Patient is stable, recovering, or improving	Yes	15
99312	Expanded problem focused	Expanded problem focused	Moderate	Responding inadequately or developed minor complication	Yes	25
99313	Detailed	Detailed	Moderate to high	Unstable or developed significant complication or new significant problem	Yes	35
Requires two of the three key components to be documented						

	The Decision Matrix for Home Services, New Patient					
Code	History	Exam	Medical Decision Making	Nature of Presenting Problem	Counseling/ Coordination of Care	Time
99341	Problem focused	Problem focused	Straightforward	Low	Yes	20
99342	Expanded problem focused	Expanded problem focused	Straightforward	Low	Yes	30
99343	Detailed	Detailed	Moderate	High	Yes	45
99344	Comprehensive	Comprehensive	Moderate	High	Yes	60
99345	Comprehensive	Comprehensive	High	Unstable problem, requires immediate attention	Yes	75

Requires all three key components to be documented

The Decision Matrix for Home Services, Established Patient						
Code	History	Exam	Medical Decision Making	Nature of Presenting Problem	Counseling/ Coordination of Care	Time
99347	Problem focused interval	Problem focused	Straightforward	Self-limited or minor	Yes	15
99348	Expanded problem focused, interval	Expanded problem focused	Low	Low to moderate	Yes	25
99349	Detailed, interval	Detailed	Moderate	Moderate to high	Yes	40
99350	Comprehensive, interval	Comprehensive	Moderate	Moderate to high	Yes	60
Requires two of the three key components to be documented						

MGMT SURG

The Decision Matrix for Domiciliary Services, New Patient

Code	History	Examination	Medical Decision Making	Nature of Presenting Problem	Counseling/ Coordination of Care	Time
99321	Problem focused	Problem focused	Straight-forward/ low	Low	Yes	N/A
99322	Expanded problem focused	Expanded problem focused	Moderate	Moderate	Yes	N/A
99323	Detailed	Detailed	High	High	Yes	N/A

Requires all three key components to be documented

MGMT SURG

The Decision Matrix for Domiciliary Services, Established Patient

Code	History	Exam	Medical Decision Making	Nature of Presenting Problem	Counseling/ Coordination of Care	Time
99331	Problem focused, interval	Problem focused	Straightforward/Low	Patient is stable, recovering, or improving	Yes	N/A
99332	Expanded problem focused, interval	Expanded problem focused	Moderate	Responding inadequately or developed minor complication	Yes	N/A
99333	Detailed, interval	Detailed	High	Unstable or developed significant complication or new significant problem	Yes	N/A

Requires two of the three key components to be documented

84

The Decision Matrix for Discharge Services

Code	Nursing Facility Discharge Day Management	Time
99238	Includes final examination, discussion of hospital stay, instructions for care, prescriptions, preparation of discharge records	30 minutes or less
99239	Includes final examination, discussion of hospital stay, instructions for care, prescriptions, preparation of discharge records	Over 30 minutes

The Decision Matrix for Preventive Medicine Services, New Patient

Initial preventive medicine service, including a comprehensive history and examination, counseling, anticipatory guidance/risk factor reduction interventions, and ordering appropriate laboratory/diagnostic procedures.

99381: Infant, under 1 year of age

99382: Early childhood, age 1–4 years

99383: Late childhood, age 5–11 years

99384: Adolescent, age 12–17 years

99385: Age 18–39 years

99386: Age 40–64 years

99387: Age 65 years and over

The Decision Matrix for Preventive Medicine Services, Established Patient

Periodic preventive medicine re-evaluation, including a comprehensive history and examination, counseling, anticipatory guidance/risk factor reduction interventions, and ordering appropriate laboratory/diagnostic procedures

99391: Infant, under 1 year of age

99392: Early childhood, age 1–4 years

99393: Late childhood, age 5–11 years

99394: Adolescent, age 12–17 years

99395: Age 18–39 years

99396: Age 40–64 years

99397: Age 65 years and over

The Decision Matrix for Prolonged Care Services, Outpatient

Code	Description	Time
99354	Prolonged physician service in the office or outpatient setting requiring direct (face-to-face) patient contact beyond the usual service	First hour
99355	Each additional 30 minutes	30

The Decision Matrix for Prolonged Care Services, Inpatient

Code	Description	Time
99356	Prolonged physician service in the office or outpatient setting requiring direct (face-to-face) patient contact beyond the usual service	First hour
99357	Each additional 30 minutes	30

The Decision Matrix for Prolonged Care Services, Without Direct Patient Contact

Code	Description	Time
99358	Prolonged physician service in the office or outpatient setting requiring direct (face-to-face) patient contact beyond the usual service	First hour
99359	Each additional 30 minutes	30

Critical Care

Critical care services are not site-specific. They can be performed in any location of the hospital. They are provided for episodes of conditions that are generally life-threatening. They are not used for in-patient days when a patient is in the Intensive Care Unit or Cardiac-Care Unit of a hospital. In these cases, the appropriate inpatient codes should be used. There is no limit to the number of critical care services that can be provided and billed each day. These services may be provided to patients under the following conditions:

- Central nervous system or circulatory system failure
- Hepatic, renal, or respiratory failure
- Severe infection
- Postoperative complications

The time providing critical care services may be spent as follows:

- Direct care to the patient
- Review of studies and test results
- Discussion of patient with other team members
- Documentation of critical care in the medical record
- Time spent with family members or patient decision makers

Critical care codes are time-based and are billed as follows:

- 99291 Critical care, first 30–74 minutes
- 99292 Critical care, each additional 30 minutes (list separately in addition to code 99291)

Examples of Billing for Critical Care Codes

Total Time Documented for Critical Care Services Provided	Billing for Critical Care
Less than 30 minutes	Use appropriate inpatient code
30–74 minutes	99291
75–104 minutes	99291 and 99292
105–134 minutes	99291 and 99292 × 2
135–164 minutes	99291 and 99292 × 3
165–194 minutes	99291 and 99292 × 4
194 minutes or more	99291 and 99292 for the length of time spent

Note: Only one physician can bill for a given hour of critical care, even though more than one physician may be involved.

Documentation Formats

Of the three currently used documentation formats, the most commonly used format is SOAP.

		Description
S	ubjective	Includes patient complaints, history of illness or injury, answers to questions about organ systems, and past, family and/or social history
O	bjective	Includes findings on examination of the patient
A	ssessment	Includes the prognosis and/or differential diagnosis of the patient and diagnostic studies
P	lan	Includes patient instructions, testing to be performed, next appointment, prescriptions, referrals

*Current Procedural Terminology © 2006 American Medical Association, All Rights Reserved.

The next most commonly used documentation format is SNOCAMP:

		Description
S	ubjective	Includes patient complaints, history of illness/injury, answers to questions about organ systems, and PFSH
N	ature of presenting problem	Includes a disease, illness, injury, symptom, or finding that relates to the chief complaint
O	bjective	Findings on patient examination
C	ounseling/ coordination of care	Patient visits where counseling constitutes more than 50% of the visit
A	ssessment	Includes prognosis and/or differential diagnosis of the patient and diagnostic studies
M	edical decision making	Complexity of the visit and physician's thought process; this component is subjective and based on 3 components: 1) number of diagnoses/management options 2) amount and/or complexity of data 3) risk of mortality/morbidity
P	lan	Includes patient instructions, tests to be performed, next appointment, Rx, referrals

The third and least common documentation format is CHEDDAR:

		Description
C	hief complaint	Includes reason for visit
H	istory	Includes history and contributing factors
E	xamination	Includes findings on examination of the patient
D	etails	Details problems and complaints of the patient
D	rug and dosage	Includes patient's current medications
A	ssessment	Includes diagnostic process and total impression
R	eturn visit	Includes information regarding the return visit and/or referral

Concurrent Care

Concurrent care is the provision of similar services to the same patient by more than one provider on the same day. When both providers bill the same diagnosis code, a claim denial may occur. If there is no documentation to support the medical necessity for the second provider, the provider who sends the claim in first gets paid, the second claim gets denied.

To eliminate this claim denial, document the need for the second provider to be involved in the patient's care. Generate a paper claim (CMS 1500 form) and attach the documentation to the form. The claim form should be completed with the appropriate CPT and ICD-9-CM codes.

Surgery Coding/Anesthesia Coding/Anesthesia

Facts:

- Anesthesia is billed using time units that equal 15 minutes per unit.
- Time begins when the physician or certified registered nurse anesthetist (CRNA) prepares the patient for induction and ends when the patient is released from anesthesia care in the recovery room.
- Time is rounded to one decimal place, when necessary.
- Time is not used when administering local medications intravenously.

Physical Status Modifiers are used to report that the anesthesia administered was complicated by the physical status of the patient.

Important facts:

- Some payers will reimburse a higher amount when these modifiers are used.
- In other cases, such as Medicare, payers do not recognize these modifiers.
- Each case is carrier-specific, and the reporting rules for the carrier must be obtained prior to submission of the claim.

Physical Status Modifiers		
Modifier	**Description**	
P1	A normal healthy patient	This modifier indicates that the patient is healthy.
P2	A patient with a mild systemic disease	This modifier indicates that the patient has some type of mild disease process, such as hypertension.

Modifier	Description	
P3	A patient with a severe systemic disease	This modifier indicates that the patient has a severe systemic disease that could affect the care of the patient. This modifier may be used with a patient who, for example, is a brittle diabetic with complications of congestive heart failure and uncontrolled hypertension.
P4	A patient with a severe systemic disease that is a threat to life	This modifier indicates that the patient has a severe disease that is a threat to life, such as a patient who has had a heart attack and now requires an angioplasty.
P5	A moribund patient who is not expected to survive without the procedure	This modifier is used for critically injured patients who require emergency surgery.
P6	A declared brain-dead patient whose organs are being removed for transplant	This modifier is used for a patient who is brain-dead and being maintained on life support while waiting for organ harvesting.

Monitored Anesthesia Care

Monitored anesthesia consists of the following:

- Preanesthesia evaluation
- Perianesthesia evaluation
- Postanesthesia evaluation
- Patient evaluation on admission and discharge from anesthesia care
- Time-based records of vital signs and level of consciousness

Medically Directed Anesthesia Services

Medically directed services occur when a physician is responsible for the direction of two, three, or four concurrent cases involving CRNAs . These medically directed services are reported using the modifier -QX.

Conscious Sedation

Conscious sedation occurs when sedation is achieved with or without the administration of an analgesic. This sedation places the patient into a lower level of consciousness, allowing for certain procedures to be carried out. Medicare does not permit these codes (99141 and 99142) to be billed separately and considers them bundled into the procedure.

HCPCS Modifiers for Anesthesia Services

Modifier	Description
AA	Anesthesia services performed personally by an anesthesiologist
AD	Medical supervision by a physician; more than four concurrent anesthesia procedures at one time
G8	Monitored anesthesia care (MAC) for deep, complex, complicated, or markedly invasive surgical procedure
G9	MAC for patient who has history of severe cardiopulmonary condition
QK	Medical direction of two, three, or four concurrent anesthesia procedures involving qualified individuals
QS	MAC service
QX	CRNA service with medical direction by a physician
QY	Anesthesiologist medically directs one CRNA
QZ	CRNA service without medical direction by a physician

*Current Procedural Terminology © 2006 American Medical Association, All Rights Reserved.

Surgery

Important Definitions

- Assistant surgeon: Assists the primary surgeon in charge of the case with a specific surgical procedure
- Cosurgeon: Two surgeons of different specialties are required for a specific surgical procedure
- Team surgery: A single procedure requires more than two different surgeons of two different specialties

Global Surgeries

Components of a global surgery package are:

- Preoperative visits
- Intraoperative services
- Complications following surgery
- Postoperative visits and pain management
- Supplies
- Miscellaneous services such as staple and suture removal, casts, splints, removal of catheters, etc.
- These items cannot be billed separately because they are considered part of the surgical package.

Services that can be billed separately are as follows:

- Separately identifiable service from the surgery (use separate diagnosis code when reporting)
- Diagnostic testing and procedures
- Second procedures that are distinct from the original procedure
- Initial consultation that prompted the decision for surgery
- History and physical performed more than 1 day before the surgery
- Reoperations due to complications
- Dialysis
- Immunosuppressive drug therapy for organ transplants
- Critical care

Modifiers used with global surgery billing

- Modifier -24
- Modifier -25
- Modifier -57
- Modifier -58
- Modifier -76
- Modifier -77
- Modifier -78
- Modifier -79

See Tab 7 for details of these modifiers.

Bilateral Surgeries

Important facts:

- If code indicates the procedure is performed on both sides of the body, then the second side cannot be billed separately
- If additional procedures are billed by the same physician on the same day, use modifier -51 (See Tab 7)

Minor Surgeries

Important facts:

- They are not usually global
- If there is a 10-day postoperative period, all surgery and postsurgery visits would be included in the global fee
- Underlying conditions can be billed separately
- The day of the procedure is not counted in the global fee period

Multiple Surgeries

Important facts:

- When two physicians of different specialties perform separate procedures during the same session, each surgeon will bill for the specific procedure performed. There is no modifier required.
- When billing a procedure code that takes one or more sessions, third-party carriers will pay one time during the global fee period.

■ When more than one procedure is performed at the same operative session, list the major procedure first, followed by the lesser procedures.

Critical Care

Critical care can be billed separately for preoperative and postoperative care when the following conditions exist:

■ Constant attention is required by the physician
■ Care is unrelated to the surgical procedure performed

Postoperative Pain

■ Bill code 62319 for the first day of pain management by continuous epidural.
■ Bill code 01996 for daily management of the epidural drug after the catheter is inserted.
■ Physician services related to patient-controlled analgesia (PCA) is included in the global fee.

Surgical Tray

Medicare can be billed for a surgical tray when certain surgical procedures are performed. Billing surgical trays with other third-party carriers is carrier-specific and requires the provider to check with each carrier individually. The code for billing surgical tray is A4550.

Components Involved in Coding From Operative Reports

An operative report consists of four main elements:
- Heading
- History or indication for surgery
- Body
- Finding

The heading consists of five major components:
- Hospital-specific information
- Patient-specific information
- Date of operation or surgery
- Specific information regarding operation
- Operation or procedure performed

Other information in the heading:
- Hardware
- Components
- Grafts
- Complications
- Drains
- Tourniquet time
- Other material left in place

Hospital-Specific Information

- Name of hospital
- Address of hospital
- Patient's medical record or other number used to track the patient
- Admission date

Patient-Specific Information

- Name, date of birth/age, sex

Date of Operation or Surgery

- Example: 11/01/2005

Specific Information Regarding Operation

- Attending surgeon: all surgeons involved should be listed, i.e., primary surgeon, cosurgeons, and assistant surgeons

- Cosurgeon
- Surgery resident, if applicable
- Surgery assistants, if applicable
- Anesthetic (general, local)
- Complications
- Estimated blood loss

Diagnosis
- Preparative diagnoses
- Postoperative diagnoses

Operation or Procedure Performed

Specific case information is inserted in this section.

History or indication for surgery

Contains a brief history why the surgery is indicated

Body (operations[s]/procedure[s] in detail)

Contains a detailed accounting of the operation(s) from start to finish

Findings

Contains a synopsis of the findings during the operation
There are other sources of documentation that could influence the coding of the operation or procedure. These documents are as follows:

- Progress notes
- Physician orders
- Pathology reports
- Discharge summary
- History and physicals
- Emergency department reports
- Ventilator management forms
- Anesthesiology forms
- Recovery room course and information
- Complications
- Ambulance services
- Consultant's reports

Surgical and Postoperative Codes

ICD-9-CM Codes

ICD-9-CM categories 996–999 contain the majority of the codes used when reporting surgical and postoperative complications. When coding an inpatient service, the condition leading to the

(Continued text on following page)

admission to the hospital is the primary code used for billing. For outpatient services, the diagnosis code that reflects the most current reason for this episode of care is primary.

The principal diagnosis is defined as the condition established "after study" to be chiefly responsible for admission of the patient to the hospital. **This definition applies to inpatient services only. It does not apply to observation care or any other type of service.**

Surgical Modifiers

Surgical modifiers used, other than those listed in the Global Surgery section of this tab, are:

- Modifier -22
- Modifier -54
- Modifier -51
- Modifier -56
- Modifier -52
- Modifier -99

Elective Surgery Notice

When **nonparticipating** providers submit a Medicare claim for an elective surgery, the patient must be presented with an elective surgery notice, which identifies the charges and their liability. This notice must be presented to the patient whenever the procedure charge is $500 or more.

Requirements for a procedure to be considered elective:

- If the surgery is postponed, there will be no damage to the patient's health
- There is no urgency for this surgery
- This surgery can be scheduled in advance

Physicians who do not participate in Medicare must provide their elective surgery patients with a fee disclosure form. This form must contain the following:

- The estimated charge (cannot be higher than the limiting charge)
- The estimated Medicare allowable charge
- The difference between the two charges
- The patient's coinsurance amount

Patient's Out-of-Pocket Expenses

The charge to the patient must not exceed 115% of the Medicare allowable amount. An example of this estimation calculation can be seen in the following table:

Description	Fee
Charge for the procedure	$1000.00
Medicare allowable amount	$550.00
Medicare approved charge (Whichever of the above fees is the lower, $1000 or $550)	$550.00
Difference between Medicare approved charge and actual charge ($1000 − $550 = $450)	$450.00
Coinsurance (20%) (20% of the Medicare approved charge: $550 × .20 = $110)	$110.00
Patient's portion of the bill if Medicare deductible has been met ($450 + $110 = $560)	**$560.00**
If the patient's Medicare deductible has not been met ($560 + $100 = $660)	**$660.00**

Integumentary System Coding

When reporting size, CPT codes are based on centimeters. The
conversion of centimeters to inches is: 2.54 cm = 1 inch.
Considerations when billing for procedures involving the skin:

- Location
  - Where is it?
- Method
  - Was it incised, excised, shaved?
- Structures
  - Did it involve only skin or did it also involve muscle?
- Depth
  - Was it deeper than the subcutaneous tissue?
- Type
  - Was it complete, partial?
- Size
  - Report using centimeters
- Number
  - How many lesions?

Incision and Drainage

Considerations when billing for incision and drainage of an abscess or cyst:

- Site
  - Arm, face, etc.
- Depth
  - Skin, soft tissue
- Method
  - Incision, puncture

Removal of Foreign Bodies

Considerations when billing for removal of foreign bodies:

- Site
  - Face, leg, hand, eye
- Depth
  - Muscle, subcutaneous tissue
- Complexity
  - Superficial, complicated

Repairs

Repair codes are used for suture lacerations from injury or procedures. If suturing is required as a result of a procedure, the reimbursement is included in that procedure code and cannot be billed separately.

Types of Repairs

Simple	Closure of a partial or full-thickness wound to the skin and subcutaneous tissues. No involvement of deep structures.
Intermediate	Closure of wounds/lacerations involving repair of one or more deeper layers of subcutaneous tissue and nonmuscle fascia along with the skin.
Complex	Closure of layered wound that requires additional work, such as scar revision, débridement, retention sutures, etc.

Considerations for repairs:

- Location
    - Foot, hand, face
- Size
    - Reported in centimeters
- Structure
    - Skin, subcutaneous tissue, muscle

Steps for Coding Wound Repairs

1. The repaired wound should be measured and recorded in centimeters, whether curved, angular, or stellate.
2. When multiple wounds are repaired, add together the lengths of those in the same classification and report as a single item. When more than one classification of wounds is repaired, list the more complicated as the primary procedure and the less complicated as the secondary procedure, using modifier -51.
3. Decontamination and/or débridement is/are considered a separate procedure only when gross contamination requires prolonged cleansing, when appreciable amounts of tissue are removed, or when débridement is carried out separately without immediate primary closure.
4. If the wound repair involves nerves, blood vessels, and/or tendons, choose codes from appropriate subsection of the Surgery section (nervous, cardiovascular, etc) for repair of these structures.

Burns

Considerations for local treatment of burns:

- Anesthesia
    - With or without
- Depth
    - Depth of burn
- Location
    - Hand, face
- Percent
    - Percent of body surface
- Size
    - Small, medium

Rule of Nines

An approximation of the area of skin burned. It divides the body into units of surface area that are divisible by nine, with the exception of the perineum. In an adult, the following are the respective percentages of the total body surface area:

Adults:

- Head and neck total for front and back: 9%
- Each upper limb total for front and back: 9%
- Thorax and abdomen front: 18%
- Thorax and abdomen back: 18%
- Perineum: 1%
- Each lower limb total for front and back: 18%

The Rule of Nines is relatively accurate for adults but not for children due to the relative disproportion of body part surface area.

Children:

- Head and neck total for front and back: 18%
- Each upper limb total for front and back: 9%
- Thorax and abdomen front: 18%
- Thorax and abdomen back: 18%
- Perineum: 1%
- Each lower limb total for front and back: 13.5%

Fracture Coding

Fracture codes include evaluation and management (E&M) services:

- E&M service the day of the fracture treatment
- Treatment of the fracture, i.e., pinning, open, closed
- Placement and removal of initial cast or splint
- Follow-up care provided

Subsequent casts can be billed separately.

Dislocations are reported by two factors:

1. The method with which they were stabilized
2. The type of manipulation used

Endoscopy Coding

There are two types of endoscopy:
1. Diagnostic   2. Therapeutic

Diagnostic Procedures	Minor Therapeutic Procedures	Major Therapeutic Procedures
Diagnostic endoscopy	Biopsy of different lesion in a different area	Removal of tumor, polyp, or lesion using hot biopsy or snare
Biopsy of the same lesion in the same area	Removal of foreign body	Ablation of tumor, polyp, or lesion by other technique
Brushing or washing to collect a specimen	Dilation	
	Removal of stent	

Miscellaneous Facts

- Use two codes when reporting the replacement of a pacemaker battery:
  - Code for the removal of the pulse generator
  - Code the insertion of the new pulse generator
- Replacement of the pacemaker within the first 2 weeks is included in the original code and cannot be billed separately
- Surgical endoscopy includes diagnostic endoscopy
- When a C-section has been performed, the physician who performed the procedure is responsible for the postpartum care
- All sleep studies include tracing, interpretation, and report
- Surgical arthroscopy includes diagnostic arthroscopy; therefore, the latter can never be billed separately
- An E&M service can be billed the same day as PT if the service is separately identifiable. The modifier -25 must be attached to the E&M service
- There are three approaches to hysterectomies:
  - Abdominal   ■ Vaginal   ■ Laparoscopic, vaginal

ANES
RAD

Radiology

Radiology billing and coding are divided into four sections:

1. Diagnostic radiology, comprising computed tomography (CT) scans, magnetic resonance imaging (MRI), and interventional radiology
2. Diagnostic ultrasound
3. Radiation oncology
4. Diagnostic and therapeutic nuclear medicine

In Current Procedural Terminology © 2006 American Medical Association, all procedures are listed by anatomical site and body system. These procedures are presented by type of service and body site. Radiation oncology is presented according to the following outline:

- Treatment planning
- Medical radiation physics
- Treatment delivery
- Treatment management

Radiology procedures are often denied coverage due to lacking medical necessity. Accurate diagnosis coding is instrumental in the reimbursement process for radiology codes. It is the responsibility of the ordering physician or physician extender (an individual whose professional level is between that of a nurse and a physician, such as a nurse practitioner or physician assistant) to provide the diagnosis when ordering a radiology procedure.

Unless the radiology service is being performed in a free-standing facility where the equipment is also owned, most radiology coding includes only the professional component. In a hospital setting, the equipment is owned by the hospital, but the interpretation is performed by the radiologist and is billed using a modifier -26, or -PC for professional component.

Component	Description	Modifier
Technical	Includes equipment, supplies, personnel (technician), costs to perform the procedure	-TC
Professional	Physician's interpretation, report; also includes costs of physician education and malpractice insurance	-26
Global	One physician provides both technical and professional components of the procedure	None

With Contrast

This phrase is used when a study is requested with the use of a contrast material for enhancement of the image. This phrase can be found with the following codes:

- CT scan
- CT angiography (CTA)
- MRI
- Magnetic resonance angiography (MRA)

Contrast material is administered via an intravenous line (within a vein), intra-articularly (within a joint), or intrathecally (within a sheath: through the theca of the spinal cord.)

CT and MRI scans are listed in the CPT book either with or without contrast. The following table shows some of these codes.

CPT Code	Description
70450	Computed tomography (CT scan) head, or brain; without contrast material
70460	With contrast material
74150	Computed tomography (CT scan) abdomen; without contrast material
74160	With contrast material

The placement of the IV line for the administration of contrast is considered part of the procedure and cannot be billed for separately.

*Current Procedural Terminology © 2006 American Medical Association, All Rights Reserved.

Positron Emission Tomography (PET) Scan

A PET scan is a diagnostic tool that is most often used to detect cancer and to examine the effects of cancer therapy by biochemical changes.

PET scans can be used in the following areas:

- Brain, heart, cancerous tumors

Emergency Department X-Rays

Medicare will pay for only one interpretation of an x-ray procedure. This interpretation fee is generally reimbursed to the radiologist for a formal written report and not the emergency department physician for review of the film. Most other carriers follow the Medicare guidelines and will not reimburse for an emergency department review.

Consultations

X-ray consultations made elsewhere must generate a written report. To bill for this consultation, use CPT code 76140.

Key Elements to Help in Radiology Coding and Billing

The following table include components of specific procedures that must be considered when choosing a code. For example, a chest x-ray is a diagnostic procedure. A chest x-ray may be a single view, frontal, code 71010; or a two-view, frontal and lateral, code 71020. It is important to read the codes carefully before assigning a code to a service or procedure. Does the diagnostic procedure have more than one view? Is it a complete or limited study? Is it with or without contrast? All of these questions must be answered to properly code a diagnostic procedure.

Diagnostic Procedures

1. Number of views
2. Complete or limited study
3. With or without contrast

Ultrasound Procedures

1. Complete or limited
2. Unilateral or bilateral
3. With or without duplex scan

Nuclear Medicine Procedures

1. Type of radionuclide
2. Amount of radionuclide
3. Limited, multiple, or whole body area
4. Single or multiple determinations
5. With or without flow
6. Qualitative or quantitative

Computed Tomography

1. With or without contrast media (type and amount)
2. Multiplaner scanning and/or reconstruction

Magnetic Resonance Imaging

1. With or without contrast media (type and amount)
2. Number of sequences

Modifiers

Modifiers used in radiology coding are -22, -26, -32, -51, -52, -53, -58, -59, -62, -66, -76, -77, -78, -79, -80, -90, -99.*

Modifier	Description	Billing Notes
-22	Unusual procedural service	■ Used rarely in radiology and, when used, requires additional documentation to support use ■ Not recognized by most carriers ■ Used with CT scans when additional views or slices are needed ■ DO NOT OVERUSE
-26	Professional component	■ Used when the physician provides an interpretation of the study; this interpretation requires a separate written and signed report; simple verbiage, such as WNL (within normal limits) or fx radius-normal, does not meet the requirement

(Continued text on following page)

Modifier	Description	Billing Notes
-32	Mandated service	■ Used when the service is mandated ■ Used rarely in radiology; sometimes used by Workers Compensation
-51	Multiple procedures	■ Use this modifier when more than one procedure is performed by the same physician on the same date on the same patient
-52	Reduced service	■ Use this modifier when a procedure is partially reduced or eliminated at the physician's direction ■ Used when a postreduction film of fracture care is taken; use the comprehensive x-ray code to identify the fracture; once the fracture has been reduced, use the comprehensive x-ray code again with modifier -52 to indicate that a reduced level of service was provided
-53	Discontinued service	■ Used when the physician chooses to terminate the procedure ■ Would be used when an x-ray procedure is discontinued because the patient is at risk ■ Use a diagnosis code that is appropriate, such as procedure not carried out because of contraindication (V64.1), procedure not carried out because of patient's election (V64.2), procedure not carried out for another reason (V64.3).

*Current Procedural Terminology © 2006 American Medical Association, All Rights Reserved.

Modifier	Description	Billing Notes
-58	Staged or related procedure or service by the same physician during the postoperative period	■ Applying this modifier to the second related procedure during a postoperative period will result in a denial of the claim ■ Cannot be used in conjunction with codes whose descriptions state that the code represents one or more services
-59	Distinct procedural service	■ This modifier indicates that the procedure was distinct or separate from the other procedure performed on the same day
-62	Two surgeons	■ Used when the skills of two physicians from two different specialties are needed to perform a procedure on a patient during the same operation ■ Cannot be used by two physicians of the same specialty
-66	Surgical team	■ Used when a complex procedure requires the services of physicians from different specialties and other highly skilled individuals ■ May be used in instances of multiple traumas, heart transplants, separation of conjoined twins
-76	Repeat procedure by same physician	■ Some carriers will not allow Radiology to use this modifier; each modifier is carrier-specific so it is always best to check with the individual carrier before using modifiers ■ It is used to indicate that the procedure had to be performed again and that this was not a duplicate billing; without using this modifier in this circumstance, the claim will be denied as a duplicate

*Current Procedural Terminology © 2006 American Medical Association, All Rights Reserved.

(Continued text on following page)

Modifier	Description	Billing Notes
-77	Repeat procedure by another physician	■ Use of this modifier is rare as a second interpretation and report are unusual in radiology ■ Add this modifier to the second service ■ Sometimes used when a physician wants a better look by using a darker density, so patient must return
-78	Return to operating for related procedure during the postoperative period	■ Used when a subsequent procedure is related to the first and requires the use of an operating room
-79	Unrelated procedure or service by the same physician during the postoperative period	■ Used when an unrelated procedure is performed by the same physician during the postoperative period of the original procedure
-99	Multiple modifiers	■ Used to report that multiple modifiers are being reported in this claim

*Current Procedural Terminology © 2006 American Medical Association, All Rights Reserved.

Diagnostic Radiology

Minimum

In the radiology section of the CPT book, the word **"minimum"** becomes a key factor in billing. This word indicates that there is no ceiling beyond what is mentioned for that particular code. See the following table for an example of this wording.

CPT Code	Description
73630	Radiologic examination, foot, complete, **minimum** three views.

If an x-ray of a left foot **contained 4 views,** the same code, **73630,** would be used.

If an x-ray of a left foot **contained 2 views**, the code **73620**, *two views,* would be used.

Transcatheter Services

Transcatheter supervision and interpretation codes include the following services:

- Contrast, angiography/venography, roadmapping, fluoroscopic guidance for the intervention
- Measurement of the vessel
- Angiography/venography completion, except for procedures through existing catheters for follow-up studies
- Diagnostic angiography/venography performed during a transcatheter therapeutic radiological and interpretative service is separately reportable, unless otherwise specified.

Diagnostic Ultrasound

Terminology

Term	Definition
A-mode	Signifies a one-dimensional ultrasonic measurement procedure
M-mode	Signifies a one-dimensional ultrasonic record amplitude and velocity of moving echo-producing structures
B scan	Signifies a two-dimensional ultrasonic scanning procedure with a two-dimensional display
Real-time scan	Signifies a two-dimensional ultrasonic scanning procedure with display of two-dimensional structure and motion with time

Doppler evaluation of vascular structures is separately reportable, unless color flow is used only for anatomic structure identification.

Radiation Oncology

Items Included in Radiation Oncology

1. Initial consultation
2. Clinical treatment planning
3. Simulation
4. Medical radiation physics
5. Dosimetry
6. Treatment devices
7. Special services
8. Clinical treatment management procedures
9. Normal follow-up care for 3 months following completion of radiation

Clinical Treatment Planning

Treatment planning for radiation oncology is a highly specialized service, which includes the following:

1. Interpretation of special testing
2. Tumor localization
3. Treatment volume determination
4. Treatment time/dosage determination
5. Choice of treatment modality
6. Determination of number and size of treatment ports
7. Selection of appropriate treatment devices

	Treatment Planning Definitions*	
1.	Simple	Planning requires a single treatment area of interest encompassed in a single port or simple parallel opposed ports with simple or no blocking
2.	Intermediate	Planning requires three or more converging ports, two separate treatment areas, multiple blocks, or special time dose constraints
3.	Complex	Planning requires highly complex blocking, custom shielding blocks, tangential ports, special wedges or compensators, three or more separate treatment areas, rotating or special beam considerations, combination of therapeutic modalities

	Therapeutic Radiology Simulation Definitions*	
1.	Simple	Simulation of a single treatment area with either a single port or parallel opposed ports; blocking is simple or may not exist
2.	Intermediate	Simulation of three or more converging ports, two separate treatment areas, multiple blocks
3.	Complex	Simulation of tangential portals, three or more treatment areas, rotation or arc therapy, complex blocking, custom shielding blocks, brachytherapy source verification, hyperthermia probe verification, or any use of contrast materials
4.	Three-dimensional	Three-dimensional reconstruction of tumor volume and surrounding reconstruction of tumor volume and surrounding critical normal tissue structures from direct CT and/or MRI scans in preparation for non coplanar or coplanar therapy; simulation uses documented three-dimensional beam's eye view volume dose displays of multiple or moving beams
	Proton Beam Definitions*	
1.	Simple	Proton treatment delivery to a single treatment area using a single nontangential or oblique port, custom block with and without compensation
2.	Intermediate	Proton treatment delivery to one or more treatment areas using two or more ports or one or more tangential or oblique ports, with custom blocks and compensators
3.	Complex	Proton treatment delivery to one or more treatment areas using two or more ports per treatment area with matching or patching fields and/or multiple isocenters, with custom blocks and compensators

Hyperthermia		
Types of Hyperthermia*		**CPT Codes**
1.	External (superficial, deep)	77600, 77605
2.	Interstitial	77610, 77615
3.	Intracavity	77620

Physics planning and interstitial insertion of temperature sensors and the use of external or interstitial heat-generating sources **are included** in the above codes. Consultations may be billed separately with the above procedures.

Clinical Brachytherapy

Brachytherapy Applications*		
1.	Simple	Application of 1–4 sources
2.	Intermediate	Application of 5–10 sources
3.	Complex	Application of more than 10 sources

*Current Procedural Terminology © 2006 American Medical Association, All Rights Reserved.

Interventional Radiology Procedures

Interventional procedures are most often performed by the same physician but may be performed by two physicians. For example, a liver biopsy may be performed by a surgeon and a radiologist. The surgeon's responsibility would be the placement of the needle and the tissue sampling. The radiologist would be responsible for performing the x-rays, dye injections, and film interpretations.

Nuclear Medicine: Diagnostic

Nuclear medicine codes do not include radium or other radioelements and should be reported separately. Nuclear medicine procedures may be performed independently or during the course of care.

Therapeutic

The administration codes for oral and intravenous administration are inclusive of the mode of administration. When reporting intra-arterial, intracavitary, and intra-articular administration, use the following codes when appropriate:

- Appropriate injection and/or procedure codes
- Imaging guidance
- Radiological supervision and interpretation codes

Basic Radiology Definitions

Term	Definition
Anteroposterior (AP)	Front to back
Anteroposterior and lateral	Two projections are included in this examination: front to back and side
Contrast material	Usually a radiopaque material that is placed into the body to enable a system or body structure to be visualized; common terms include nonionic and low osmolar contrast medial (LOCM), ionic and high osmolar contrast media (HOCM), barium, and gadolinium
Decubitus (DEC)	Patient lying on the side
Frontal	Face forward
Lateral (LAT)	Side view
Modality	A form of imaging, including x-ray, fluoroscopy, ultrasound, nuclear medicine, duplex Doppler, CT, and MRI
Oblique (OBL)	Oblique view of the object being x-rayed
Posteroanterior (PA)	Back to front
Real-time	Immediate imaging, usually in movement
Stent	Tube providing support in a body cavity or lumen
Subtraction	The removal of an overlying structure to better visualize the structure in question; this is done in a series by imposing one x-ray on top of another

(Continued text on following page)

Term	Definition
Tomogram	A specialized type of x-ray imaging that provides slices through a body structure in order to obliterate overlying structures; commonly performed for studies of the kidneys and temporomandibular joint (TMJ)

Laboratory

Modifiers

Modifiers used in pathology coding are -22, -26, -32, -52, -53, -59, -90, -91. Laboratory and pathology studies cover the following areas:

- Organ panels
- Urinalysis
- Chemistry
- Hematology
- Blood banking
- Drug testing
- Cytopathology
- Surgical pathology

Organ panels consist of various components that are generally ordered together. An example can be seen in the following basic metabolic panel:

Test	CPT Code*
Calcium	82310
Carbon dioxide	82374
Chloride	82435
Creatinine	82565
Glucose	82947
Potassium	84132
Sodium	84295
Urea nitrogen	84520

*Current Procedural Terminology © 2006 American Medical Association, All Rights Reserved.

The above tests, as with other panels, are components of the basic metabolic panel and would be billed using CPT code 80048. Billing all of the above codes individually would be unbundling (description of this term is in Tab 5) and therefore would be considered a matter of fraud and abuse. If only two of the above tests are ordered, obviously only the two individual codes would be billed.

Other organ panels are:

Panel	CPT Code*
General heal panel	80050
Electrolyt panel	80051
Comprehensive metabolic panel	80053
Obstetric panel	80055
Lipid panel	80061
Renal function panel	80069
Acute hepatitis panel	80074
Hepatic function panel	80076

In addition to the widely ordered panels above, other common tests are:

Test	CPT Code*
Urinalysis, by dip stick, non-automated, with microscopy	81000
Urinalysis, by dip stick, automated, with microscopy	81001
Urinalysis, by dip stick, non-automated, without microscopy	81002
Urinalysis, by dip stick, automated, without microscopy	81003
Cholesterol, total	82465
Triglycerides	84478
Glucose, quantitative, except reagent strip	82947
Glucose, blood, reagent strip	82948
Glucose tolerance test, 3 specimens	82951
Beyond 3 specimens	82952

(Continued text on following page)

Test	CPT Code*
Glucose, monitoring device for home use	82962
Prostate-specific antigen (PSA)	84152
Thyroid stimulating hormone (TSH)	84443
Gonadotropin, chorionic, quantitative (HCG)	84702
Blood count, automated diff with WBC	85004
Complete blood count (CBC), automated, with automated diff. Includes Hgb, Hct, RBC, WBC, and platelet count	85025
Complete blood count (CBC) without diff.	85027
Prothrombin time	85610
Partial thromboplastin (PTT)	85730
Urine culture, bacterial, quantitative colony count	87086
Sensitivity studies, antibiotic disk method, per plate (12 fewer discs)	87184

Surgical Pathology

Surgical pathology codes include accession, examination, and report. There are six levels of surgical pathology codes.

Level	Definition and Examples of Level*	CPT Code
I	**Surgical pathology, gross exam**	**88300**
II	**Surgical pathology, gross and microscopic exam**	**88302**
	■ Appendix	
	■ Skin, plastic repair	
	■ Vas deferens, sterilization	
III	**Surgical pathology, gross and microscopic exam**	**88304**
	■ Carpal tunnel tissue	

*Current Procedural Terminology © 2006 American Medical Association, All Rights Reserved.

Level	Definition and Examples of Level*	CPT Code
	■ Gallbladder	
	■ Tonsils	
IV	**Surgical pathology, gross and microscopic exam**	88305
	■ Colon biopsy	
	■ Joint resection	
	■ Stomach biopsy	
V	**Surgical pathology, gross and microscopic exam**	88307
	■ Breast, mastectomy – partial/simple	
	■ Cervix, conization	
	■ Liver biopsy – needle/wedge	
VI	**Surgical pathology, gross and microscopic exam**	88309
	■ Colon, total resection	
	■ Prostate, radical resection	
	■ Soft tissue tumor, extensive resection	

Collection of Specimen*

Description	CPT Code
1. Venipuncture, routine collection of venous blood	36415
2. Venipuncture, routine collection of venous blood, Medicare patient	G0001
3. Collection of capillary blood specimen (heel, finger, ear)	36416

*Current Procedural Terminology © 2006 American Medical Association, All Rights Reserved.

Unbundling

The process of coding integral services separately from a procedure is called unbundling. If the component is considered part of the bundled service, it cannot be coded separately. For example, CPT code 93000 is a code for Electrocardiogram, routine ECG, with at least 12 leads, with interpretation and report. If codes 93005 (ECG tracing only, without interpretation and report) and 93010 (ECG with interpretation and report only) were billed together, it would be considered unbundling, as both elements are found in the all-inclusive CPT code of 93000.

Add-On Codes

There are codes that are performed in addition to the main CPT code.
Add-On Code Facts:

- These codes are called Add-on codes.
- They are not reported with the modifier -51 for multiple procedures as other CPT codes would be.
- They cannot be billed by themselves.
- Add-on codes are identified by wording that designates them as add-on codes.

Examples:

Primary Code*	Description	Add-On Code	Description
96408	Chemotherapy administration, intravenous; push technique	96412	Infusion technique, 1 to 8 hours, each additional hour (list separately in addition to code for primary procedure)
92607	Evaluation for prescription for speech-generating augmentative and alternative communication device, face-to-face with the patient; first hour	92608	Each additional 30 minutes (list separately in addition to code for primary procedure)

*Current Procedural Terminology © 2006 American Medical Association, All Rights Reserved.

There are instances where more than one add-on code is used. See the following table:

Primary Code*	Add-On Code	Description	Second Add-On Code	Description
Any outpatient evaluation and management code (e.g., 99201–99205, 99211–99215, 99241–99245)	99354	Prolonged physician service in the office or other outpatient setting requiring direct (face-to-face) patient contact beyond the usual service (e.g., prolonged care and treatment of an acute asthmatic patient in an outpatient setting); first hour (list separately in addition to code for office or other outpatient Evaluation and Management code)	99355	Each additional 30 minutes (list separately in addition to code for primary procedure)

*Current Procedural Terminology © 2006 American Medical Association, All Rights Reserved.

Multiple Procedure/Services

Certain procedures can be reported separately without the risk of unbundling. For example, a patient hospitalized for a mental condition can receive interactive psychotherapy in conjunction with an Evaluation and Management code. Both the psychotherapy code and the Evaluation and Management codes would be billed for that date of service.

Separate Procedures

Any code that is designated as a "separate procedure" cannot be billed in addition to the code for the comprehensive procedure. If a code listed as "separate procedure" is coded independent of any other procedure, it can then be billed.

Injections

Injections of immune globulins require the CPT code for the actual Immune Globulin serum and a CPT code for the administration of the injection. Immune globulin codes go from 90281 to 90399 for the serum. They should be reported with the appropriate delivery code. These codes go from 90780 to 90784. A description of codes 90780 and 90781 can be found in the following section. Vaccines and toxoids are reported using codes 90476 to 90748. Descriptions of codes 90782 to 90784 are described in the following table:

CPT Code*	Description
90782	Therapeutic, prophylactic, or diagnostic injection (specify material injected); subcutaneous or intramuscular
90783	■ Intra-arterial
90784	■ Intravenous

*Current Procedural Terminology © 2006 American Medical Association, All Rights Reserved.

Administration codes are also used for reporting injections of antibiotics.

CPT Code*	Description
90788	Intramuscular injection of antibiotic is used in addition to reporting the drug (antibiotic).

Immunization administration codes for vaccines are reported using the following administration codes:

CPT Code*	Description
90465	Immunization administration under 8 years old (includes percutaneous, intradermal, subcutaneous, or intramuscular) when the physician counsels the patients; first injection (single or combination vaccine/toxoid), per day
90466	■ Each additional injection (single or combination vaccine/toxoid) per day; list separately in addition to code for primary procedure
90467	Immunization administration under 8 years old (includes intranasal or oral routes of administration) when the physician counsels the patient; first administration (single or combination vaccine/toxoid), per day
90468	■ Each additional administration (single or combination vaccine/toxoid) per day; list separately in addition to code for primary procedure
90471	Immunization administration (includes percutaneous, intradermal, subcutaneous, or intramuscular), one vaccine (single or combination vaccine/toxoid)

(Continued text on following page)

CPT Code*	Description
90472	■ Each additional vaccine (single or combination vaccine/toxoid); list separately in addition to code for primary procedure
90473	Immunization administration by intranasal or oral route; one vaccine (single or combination vaccine/toxoid)
90474	■ Each additional vaccine (single or combination vaccine/toxoid); list separately in addition to code for primary procedure

Therapeutic, Diagnostic Infusions (Excludes Chemotherapy)

CPT codes 90780 and 90781 are used to report prolonged intravenous injections. They are not used for billing of the following services:

- Intradermal
- Subcutaneous
- Intramuscular
- Routine intravenous (IV)

Choose the appropriate code based on time.

CPT Code*	Description	Time
90780	IV infusion for therapy/diagnosis, administered by physician or under direct supervision of physician	Up to 1 hour
90781	■ Each additional hour up to 8 hours; list separately in addition to the code for the primary procedure	2–8 hours

*Current Procedural Terminology © 2006 American Medical Association, All Rights Reserved.

Psychiatry

Billing codes* for psychiatry evaluation services include:
90801–90802: Psychiatric diagnostic interview examinations
Office or Outpatient

90804–90809: Insight oriented, behavior modifying and/or
supportive psychotherapy
90810–90815: Interactive psychotherapy
Inpatient Hospital, Partial Hospital, or Residential Care Facility
90816–90822: Insight oriented, behavior modifying and/or
supportive psychotherapy
90823–90829: Interactive psychotherapy
90845–90857: Other psychotherapy
90862–90899: Other psychiatric services or procedures

Guide to coding psychiatric services:

- Psychiatric diagnostic interviews must include history, mental status, and a disposition
- Interactive psychiatric diagnostic interviews are generally provided to children; they use physical aids and nonverbal communication to overcome barriers between the patient and the clinician due to language skills that have either been lost or have not yet developed
- Psychiatric therapeutic services are found in two categories:
  - Interactive psychotherapy
  - Insight oriented behavior modifying and/or supportive psychotherapy
- Some patients receive psychotherapy only, and others receive Evaluation and Management services (see Tab 2) in addition.
- Psychotherapy codes are chosen based on the type of psychotherapy, the place of service, face-to-face time spent with the patient, and whether an E&M code is performed on the same day.
- Medicare **will not** accept psychiatric therapy codes 90804–90829 billed on the same day as an E&M code.

---

*Current Procedural Terminology © 2006 American Medical Association, All Rights Reserved.

Physical Medicine and Rehabilitation

Important facts:

- Medicare patients and many other carriers require a written plan of care before the patient begins physical therapy
- Some codes are time-based and therefore require the documentation of time to be billable.

Some examples of commonly used physical therapy codes are:

CPT Code*	Description
97001	Physical therapy evaluation
97002	Physical therapy re-evaluation
97003	Occupational therapy evaluation
97004	Occupational therapy re-evaluation
97010	Application of a modality to one or more areas (hot or cold packs)
97012	■ Traction, mechanical
97014	■ Electrical stimulation (unattended)
97022	■ Whirlpool
97026	■ Infrared
97028	■ Ultraviolet
97032	Application of a modality to one or more areas; electrical stimulation (manual), each 15 minutes
97033	■ Iontophoresis, each 15 minutes
97035	■ Ultrasound, each 15 minutes
97110	Therapeutic procedure, one or more areas, each 15 minutes; therapeutic exercises to develop strength and endurance, range of motion, and flexibility

*Current Procedural Terminology © 2006 American Medical Association, All Rights Reserved.

CPT Code*	Description
97116	■ Gait training (includes stair-climbing)
97124	■ Massage, including effleurage, petrissage, and tapotement (stroking, compression, percussion)
97140	Manual therapy techniques (e.g., mobilization/ manipulation, manual lymphatic drainage, manual traction), one or more regions, each 15 minutes
97150	Therapeutic procedure(s), group (2 or more individuals)

Gastroenterology

Gastroenterology is the study of the stomach and intestine and diseases associated with them. Following is a select list of the most commonly used codes for these services. A complete listing can be found in the Medicine section of the CPT book under subsection Gastroenterology.

CPT Code*	Description
91000	Esophageal intubation and collection of washings for cytology, including preparation of specimens (separate procedure)
91010	Esophageal motility
91105	Gastric intubation, and aspiration or lavage for treatment (for ingested poisons)

Gastroenterology Surgical Codes

There are many other gastroenterology codes listed in the Surgery section of the CPT book. Some of the most commonly used codes are:

Important definitions

■ Sigmoidoscopy: the examination of the entire rectum, sigmoid colon and may include examination of a portion of the descending colon.

■ Colonoscopy: the examination of the entire colon, from the rectum to the cecum, and may include the examination of the terminal ileum.

CPT Code*	Description
43235	Upper gastrointestinal endoscopy including esophagus, stomach, and either the duodenum and/or jejunum as appropriate; diagnostic, with or without collection of specimens by brushing or washing (separate procedure)
43239	■ With biopsy, single or multiple
43243	■ With injection sclerosis of esophageal and/or gastric varices
43246	■ With directed placement of percutaneous gastrostomy tube
43260	Endoscopic retrograde cholangiopancreatography (ERCP)
43261	■ With biopsy, single or multiple
43262	■ With sphincterotomy/papillotomy
43264	■ With endoscopic retrograde removal of calculus from biliary and/or pancreatic ducts

There is sometimes confusion between the two procedures and codes explained above. It is important to read the procedural report carefully to establish the completeness of the examination.

*Current Procedural Terminology © 2006 American Medical Association, All Rights Reserved.

CPT Code*	Description
45330	Sigmoidoscopy, flexible; diagnostic, with or without collection of specimen(s) by brushing or washing (separate procedure)
45331	■ With biopsy, single or multiple
45333	■ With removal of tumor(s), polyp(s), or other lesion(s) by hot biopsy forceps or bipolar cautery
45338	■ With removal of tumor(s), polyp(s), or other lesion(s) by snare technique
45378	Colonoscopy, flexible, proximal to splenic flexure; diagnostic, with or without collection of specimen(s) by brushing or washing, with or without colon decompression (separate procedure)
45380	■ With biopsy, single or multiple
45382	■ With control of bleeding (e.g., injection, bipolar cautery, unipolar cautery, laser, heater probe, stapler, plasma coagulator)
45383	■ With ablation of tumor(s), polyp(s), or other lesion(s) not amenable to removal by hot biopsy forceps, bipolar cautery, or snare technique
45384	■ With removal of tumor(s), polyp(s), or other lesion(s) by hot biopsy forceps or bipolar cautery
45385	■ With removal of tumor(s), polyp(s), or other lesion(s) by snare technique

*Current Procedural Terminology © 2006 American Medical Association, All Rights Reserved.

Ophthalmology

Ophthalmology is the study of the eye: its anatomy, physiology, and pathology. Following is a select list of the most commonly used codes for these services. A complete listing can be found in the Medicine section of the CPT book under subsection Ophthalmology.

There are three types of ophthalmology services:

(Continued text on following page)

Type	Description
Intermediate	Evaluation of a new or existing condition complicated with a new diagnostic or management problem not necessarily relating to the primary diagnosis, including history, general medical observation, external ocular and adnexal examination and other diagnostic procedures as indicated; may include the use of mydriasis for ophthalmoscopy
Comprehensive	Evaluation of the complete visual system; consists of a single service entity but need not be performed at one session; includes history, general medical observation, external and ophthalmoscopic examinations, gross visual fields, and basic sensorimotor examination; it often includes, as indicated, biomicroscopy, examination with cycloplegia or mydriasis and tonometry; includes initiation of diagnostic and treatment programs
Special	Services in which a special evaluation of part of the visual system is made, which goes beyond the services included under the general ophthalmological services

CPT Code*	Description
92002	Ophthalmological service: medical examination and evaluation with initiation of diagnostic and treatment program; intermediate, new patient
92004	■ Comprehensive, new patient, one or more visits
92012	Ophthalmological service: medical examination and evaluation with initiation or continuation of diagnostic and treatment program; intermediate, established patient

*Current Procedural Terminology © 2006 American Medical Association, All Rights Reserved.

CPT Code*	Description
92014	■ Comprehensive, established patient, one or more visits

Codes used for office visits can be either the Ophthalmology codes or the Evaluation and Management codes; it is the physician's choice.

Biofeedback

There are two codes used to report biofeedback services. These codes may require preauthorization by the carrier.

CPT Code*	Description
90901	Biofeedback training by any modality
90911	Biofeedback training, perineal muscles, anorectal or urethral sphincter, including EMG and/or manometry

Dialysis

End-Stage Renal Disease (ESRD)

ESRD services are outpatient services and are reported with the following codes:

CPT Code*	Description
90918–90921	ESRD-related services per full month
90922–90925	ESRD-related services (less than a full month), per day

Guide to Reporting ESRD
- The various levels are age-specific
- These codes are not billable with hospitalization codes
- Codes 90918–90921 are used to report consecutive services
- Codes 90922–90925 are used to report services that are not performed consecutively during the month
- Each month is considered to be 30 days
- Procedures for other medical problems and complications unrelated to ESRD are not included in the monthly ESRD service and are reported separately

Hemodialysis

Hemodialysis codes are inpatient codes used to report hemodialysis procedures in addition to E&M codes for the same day. Services are reported with the following codes:

CPT Code*	Description
90935	Hemodialysis procedure with single physician evaluation
90937	Hemodialysis procedure requiring repeated evaluations with or without substantial revision of the dialysis prescription
90939	Hemodialysis access flow study to determine blood flow in grafts and arteriovenous fistulae by an indicator dilution method, hook-up; transcutaneous measurement and disconnection
90940	■ Measurement and disconnection

*Current Procedural Terminology © 2006 American Medical Association, All Rights Reserved.

Miscellaneous Dialysis Procedures

There are dialysis procedures other than hemodialysis. These codes are reported using CPT codes 90945 and 90947.

CPT Code*	Description
90945	Dialysis procedure other than hemodialysis (e.g., peritoneal dialysis, hemofiltration, or other continuous renal replacement therapies), with single physician evaluation
90947	Dialysis procedure other than hemodialysis (e.g., peritoneal dialysis, hemofiltration, or other continuous renal replacement therapies) requiring repeated physician evaluations, with or without substantial revision of dialysis prescription
90997	Hemoperfusion, e.g., with activated charcoal or resin

*Current Procedural Terminology © 2006 American Medical Association, All Rights Reserved.

Dialysis Training

Dialysis training is reported using CPT codes 90989–90993. Code 90989 is used to report the completion of the dialysis training course. Code 90993 is used to report training per session.

Otorhinolaryngologic Services

Otorhinolaryngology is the study of the ear, nose, and throat. Following is a select list of the most commonly used codes for these services. A complete listing can be found in the Medicine section of the CPT book under subsection Special Otorhinolaryngologic Services.

Diagnostic procedures are reported as part of the office visit code and cannot be billed separately. This includes such tests as otoscopy, rhinoscopy, tuning fork test, and whispered voice.

CPT Code*	Description
92506	Evaluation of speech, language, voice, communication, auditory processing, and/or aural rehabilitation status
92507	Treatment of speech, language, voice, communication, auditory processing, and/or aural rehabilitation status

Cardiovascular Services

Cardiology is the study of the heart and its functions. Following is a select list of most commonly used cardiology codes. A complete listing can be found in the Medicine section of the CPT book under subsection Cardiovascular.

Important Definitions

- Echocardiography: Echocardiography includes obtaining ultrasonic signals from the heart and great arteries, with two-dimensional image and/or Doppler ultrasonic signal documentation, and interpretation and report.
- Cardiac catheterization: Cardiac catheterization is a diagnostic medical procedure that includes introduction, positioning and repositioning of catheter(s), when necessary, recording of intracardiac and intravascular pressure, obtaining blood samples for measurement of blood gases or dilution curves and cardiac output measurements (Fick or other method, with or without rest and exercise and/or studies) with or without electrode catheter placement, final evaluation and report of procedure.

CPT Code*	Description
92950	Cardiopulmonary resuscitation (CPR) (cardiac arrest)
92982	Percutaneous transluminal coronary balloon angioplasty; single vessel
93000	Electrocardiogram, routine ECG, with at least 12 leads; with interpretation and report

CPT Code*	Description
93005	■ Tracing only, without interpretation and report
93010	■ Interpretation and report only
93015	Cardiovascular stress test using maximal or submaximal treadmill or bicycle, continuous electrocardiographic monitoring, and/or pharmacological stress; with physician supervision, with interpretation and report
93040	Rhythm ECG, one to three leads; with interpretation and report
93224	Electrocardiographic monitoring for 24 hours by continuous original ECG waveform recording and storage, with visual superimposition scanning; includes recording, scanning analysis with report, physician review and interpretation
93307	Echocardiography, transthoracic, real-time with image documentation (2D) with or without M-mode recording; complete
93320	Copper echocardiography, pulsed wave and/or continuous wave with spectral display (list separately in addition to codes for echocardiographic imaging); complete
93325	Doppler echocardiography color flow velocity mapping (list separately in addition to codes for echocardiography)
93350	Echocardiography, transthoracic, real-time with image documentation (2D) with or without M-mode recording; during rest and cardiovascular stress test using treadmill, bicycle exercise and/or pharmacologically induced stress, with interpretation and report
93501	Right heart catheterization
93510	Left heart catheterization

Electrocardiograms can be called either ECGs or EKGs.
*Current Procedural Terminology © 2006 American Medical Association, All Rights Reserved.

Pulmonary

Pulmonary medicine is the study of the lungs and/or the pulmonary artery. Following is a select list of most commonly used pulmonary codes. A complete listing can be found in the Medicine section of the CPT book under subsection Pulmonary.

CPT Code*	Description
94010	Spirometry, including graphic record, total and timed vital capacity, expiratory flow rate measurement(s), with or without maximal voluntary ventilation
94060	Bronchospasm evaluation: Spirometry as in 94010, before and after bronchodilator (aerosol or parenteral)
94150	Vital capacity, total (separate procedure)
94656	Ventilation assist and management, initiation of pressure volume preset ventilators for assisted or controlled breathing, first day
94657	■ Subsequent days
94660	Continuous positive airway pressure ventilation (CPAP), initiation and management
94664	Demonstration and/or evaluation of patient utilization of an aerosol generator, nebulizer, metered dose inhaler or IPPB device

*Current Procedural Terminology © 2006 American Medical Association, All Rights Reserved.

Allergy and Clinical Immunology

Allergy sensitivity testing is the performance and evaluation of selective cutaneous and mucous membrane tests in correlation with the history, physical examination, and other observations of the patient. Immunology is the parenteral administration of allergenic extracts as antigens at periodic intervals, usually in increasing amounts to a dosage that is maintained as maintenance therapy. A complete listing of codes can be found in the Medicine section of the CPT book under subsection Allergy and Clinical Immunology.

Important Billing and Coding Facts:

- Professional services (Evaluation and Management codes) are included in CPT codes 95115–95199, which are the allergen immunotherapy codes
- Evaluation and Management codes can be used only if there is a separate and identifiable service being performed on the same date; use modifier -25 with the Evaluation and Management code should this occur
- Codes 95115 and 95117 do not include the extract itself, only administration of the allergy injection
- Codes 95120 to 95134 include both the administration of the injection and the extract; these are referred to as complete service codes, as they also include the preparation, antigen, supplies, and observation of the patient after injection
- Code number of allergens correctly; for example:
  - 95130: Single stinging insect venom
  - 95131: Two stinging insect venoms
  - 95132: Three stinging insect venoms

Neurology and Neuromuscular Procedures

Neurology is the study of the nervous system. Following is a select list of most commonly used neurology codes. A complete listing can be found in the Medicine section of the CPT book under Neurology and Neuromuscular Procedures.

Important Billing and Coding Facts:
- Hyperventilation and phonic stimulation are included in codes 95812–95822 and cannot be billed separately
- EEG codes are time-based codes and must be chosen correctly based on time of monitoring
- Electromyography and nerve conduction tests are based on the number of extremities tested

CPT Codes*	Description
95812	Electroencephalogram (EEG) extended monitoring; 41–60 minutes
95813	■ Greater than 1 hour
95816	EEG including recording awake and drowsy
95819	■ Including awake and asleep
95860	Needle electromyography; one extremity with or without related paraspinal areas
95861	■ Two extremities with or without related paraspinal areas
95863	■ Three extremities with or without related paraspinal areas
95864	■ Four extremities with or without related paraspinal areas
95900	Nerve conduction, amplitude, and latency/velocity study, each nerve; motor, without F-wave study
95903	■ Motor, with F-wave study
95904	■ Sensory

*Current Procedural Terminology © 2006 American Medical Association, All Rights Reserved.

Chemotherapy

Chemotherapy is the treatment of various diseases by using chemical agents. Following is a select list of the most commonly used Chemotherapy codes. A complete listing can be found in the Medicine section of the CPT book under Chemotherapy.

Important Facts:

- Evaluation and Management codes can be billed with Chemotherapy procedures when warranted
- Preparation of the chemotherapy is included in the administration code
- When chemotherapy is delivered by different techniques, each codes should be billed separately by method of delivery

CPT Code*	Description
96400	Chemotherapy administration, subcutaneous or intramuscular, with or without local anesthesia
96408	Chemotherapy administration, intravenous; push technique
96410	■ Infusion technique, up to 1 hour
96412	■ Infusion technique, 1 to 8 hours, each additional hour (list separately in addition to code for primary procedure)
96420	Chemotherapy administration, intra-arterial push technique
96422	■ Infusion technique, up to 1 hour
96423	■ Infusion technique, 1 to 8 hours, each additional hour (list separately in addition to code for primary procedure)
96520	Refilling and maintenance of portable pump
96530	Refilling and maintenance of implantable pump or reservoir for drug delivery, systemic (e.g., intravenous, intra-arterial)

Sedation With or Without Analgesia (Conscious Sedation)

Conscious sedation is used to provide a medically controlled state of depressed consciousness while maintaining the patient's airway, protective reflexes, and ability to respond to stimulation or verbal commands.

Important Facts:
■ Pre- and postsedation evaluations are included in these codes and cannot be billed separately.
■ Administration of the drug and monitoring of the cardiorespiratory function are also included in these codes and cannot be billed separately.

CPT Code*	Description
99141	Sedation with or without analgesia, intravenous, intramuscular, or inhalation
99142	■ Oral, rectal, and/or intranasal

*Current Procedural Terminology © 2006 American Medical Association, All Rights Reserved.

(ICD-9-CM)

The International Classification of Diseases, 9th edition, Clinical Modifications (ICD-9-CM) is the coding system used to report the diagnosis or condition of the patient. This system takes a description of the patient's condition, illness, or injury, and translates it into numerical and alphanumerical format. The ICD-9-CM manual is published in the Spring and Fall each year. To ensure that the codes billed are accurate, it is necessary to purchase a new manual each year. These codes provide the medical necessity for the service or procedure that was performed.

Dx Codes = Medical Necessity = Reimbursement

Three Volumes of ICD-9-CM

Volume 1	The most specific information about the conditions, diseases, and injuries
Volume 2	An alphabetic listing of Volume 1
Volume 3	Information reserved for hospital use

Volume One

A listing of the chapters of Volume 1 of the ICD-9-CM manual is in the following table:

Chapter	Title	Diagnosis Codes
1	Infectious and Parasitic Diseases	Codes 001–139
2	Neoplasms	Codes 140–239
3	Endocrine, Nutritional and Metabolic Diseases, and Immunity Disorders	Codes 240–279

(Continued text on following page)

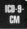
ICD-9-CM

Chapter	Title	Diagnosis Codes
4	Diseases of the Blood and Blood-Forming Organs	Codes 280–289
5	Mental Disorders	Codes 290–319
6	Diseases of the Nervous System and Sense Organs	Codes 320–389
7	Diseases of the Circulatory System	Codes 390–459
8	Diseases of the Respiratory System	Codes 460–519
9	Diseases of the Digestive System	Codes 520–579
10	Diseases of the Genitourinary System	Codes 580–629
11	Complications of Pregnancy, Childbirth, and the Puerperium (the period of confinement after labor)	Codes 630–677
12	Diseases of the Skin and Subcutaneous Tissue	Codes 680–709
13	Diseases of the Musculoskeletal System and Connective Tissue	Codes 710–739
14	Congenital Anomalies	Codes 740–759
15	Certain Conditions Originating in the Perinatal Period (period shortly before and after birth)	Codes 760–779
16	Symptoms, Signs, and Ill-Defined Conditions	Codes 780–799
17	Injury and Poisoning	Codes 800–999

Supplemental Chapters	Diagnosis Codes
V Codes: Supplemental Classification of Factors Influencing Health Status and Contact with Health Services	Codes V01-V83
E Codes: Supplemental Classification of External Causes of Injury and Poisoning	Codes E800–E999

Appendices	Title
A	Morphology of Neoplasms (M Codes)
B	Glossary of Mental Disorders
C	Classification of Drugs by American Hospital Formulary Service List Number and Their ICD-9-CM Equivalents
D	Classification of Industrial Accidents According to Agency
E	Three-Digit Categories

Volume Two	
Three Sections	
1	Index to Diseases and Injuries
2	Table of Drugs and Chemicals
3	Alphabetic Index to External Causes of Injuries and Poisonings

Easy Diagnosis Coding

Steps	Rules
1	Determine the main term that best describes the condition or symptom of the patient
2	Use Volume 2 to look up the main term; this volume is alphabetized
3	Read any cross-references such as "*see also*" and go to that category
4	Read all subterms and explanations; refer to *indented* terms under the main term to obtain further clarification.
5	Check the code listed in Volume 2 against the tabular listing in Volume 1
6	Review all instructions and notes in Volume 1 to be sure the code selected is accurate

Coding Conventions

Convention	Definition/Example
Typeface	**Bold type** indicates main terms and codes in Volume 1. EXAMPLE: CONVULSIONS **Brain 780.39** **Febrile 780.31**
Italics	This type indicates categories that cannot be reported as a primary diagnosis code. This *type* is also used for identifying exclusion notes. Example: 250 Diabetes Mellitus *Excludes gestational diabetes (648.8)*

Convention	Definition/Example
[Brackets]	These are used to enclose synonyms, alternative terminology, or explanatory phrases. Example: 482.2 Pneumonia due to *Haemophilus influenzae* [*H. influenzae*]
(Parentheses)	These are used to enclose supplementary words that may be present in the description. Example: 198.4 Other parts of nervous system Meninges (cerebral) (spinal)
Colons:	These are used in the tabular listing after an incomplete term that needs a modifier to make it assignable. Example: 021.1 Enteric tularemia Tularemia: cryptogenic intestinal
Braces }	These enclose a series of terms, each of which is modified by the statement appearing to the right of the brace. Example: 560.2 Volvulus Knotting Strangulation } of intestine, bowel or colon

ICD-10

The following list contains changes that occurred between the 9th revision of the ICD code book (ICD-9-CM) and the 10th revision. Volume I is a tabular listing that contains alphanumeric codes. Volume II is an instructional manual, which provides rules and regulations for mortality and morbidity coding. Volume III is the alphabetic index, which provides the index to all the codes listed in Volume I. The ICD-10 contains more descriptions.

(Continued text on following page)

ICD-9-CM

ICD-9-CM	ICD-10
Old Title: International Classification of Diseases, 9th Revision, Clinical Modifications	New Title: International Statistical Classification of Diseases and Related Health Problems
Contains a chapter titled Diseases of the Nervous System and Sense Organs	Splits the chapter among the following chapters: ■ Diseases of the Nervous System ■ Diseases of the Eye and Adnexa ■ Diseases of the Ear and Mastoid Process
Contains a chapter titled Mental Disorders	Renames this chapter Mental and Behavioral Disorders
Supplement: Classification of Factors Influencing Health Status and Contact with Health Services (V codes)	Becomes a chapter and is no longer a supplement to the code book
Supplement: Classification of External Causes of Injury and Poisoning (E codes)	Becomes a chapter and is no longer a supplement to the code book
Contains codes that require 4 and 5 digits	Contains codes that require 4, 5, and 6 digits

Many other changes have been made to the descriptions throughout the book. This book was published in 1994 and is currently used in Europe. It is expected to be implemented in the United States in 2007.

V Codes

V codes describe circumstances surrounding a patient's health status and identify reasons for medial treatment other than for a disease process or injury.

Three Categories
1. Problem-Oriented
2. Service-Oriented
3. Fact-Oriented

V codes can be used as primary codes in certain instances; for examples, see the following table:

Scenario	Code
Patient presents for removal of cast	V54.8
Patient presents for preoperative clearance	V72.8__
Patient presents for chemotherapy	V58.1

Problem-Oriented

A problem-oriented V code identifies a factor that may affect the patient but that is not an injury or an illness. Examples of problem oriented V codes are:

- V76.11: Special screening mammogram for high-risk patients
- V69.1: Inappropriate diet and eating habits

Service-Oriented

A service-oriented V code identifies that a service was an examination, therapy, ancillary service, or aftercare. It identifies a patient who is not currently sick but who is looking for medical services for another reason. Examples of service-oriented V codes are:

- V67.2: Follow-up examination following cancer chemotherapy
- V58.3: Removal of sutures

Fact-Oriented

A fact-oriented V code simply states a fact. Examples of fact-oriented V codes are:

- V27.2: Outcome of delivery; twins, both live-born
- V02.6: Viral hepatitis

E Codes

E codes are used to establish medical necessity, identify causes of injury and poisoning, and identify medications.

1. Can never be primary codes
2. Do not affect the amount of reimbursement
3. Can speed up the reimbursement process by providing additional information to the insurance payor
4. Child abuse takes precedent over all other E codes
5. Cataclysmic events take priority over all other E codes, except for child abuse
6. Transportation accidents take priority over all other E codes, except cataclysmic events and abuse

Examples of E codes are:

- E884.0: Fall from playground equipment
- E917.0: Struck accidentally by object or persons in sports
- E901: Excessive cold

Late Effect Codes

Two types of Late Effect codes:

- General
- Injury-related

Late Effect codes should be the primary diagnosis when it is the primary reason for the visit. To use Late Effect codes, first code the condition of the late effect, then code the late effect. For example:

- 012.22: Isolated tracheal tuberculosis, bacterial examination unknown
- 137.0: Late effects of respiratory tuberculosis

General Late Effect Codes

These codes describe a residual condition produced after the acute phase of an illness (usually 1 year or more). Examples of these codes are:

- 137.: Late effects of tuberculosis
- 438.: Late effects of cerebrovascular accident

Late Effects of Injuries, Poisonings, Toxic Effects, and Other External Causes

These codes can be used to indicate a cause of "late effect" in which the cause is classified elsewhere. These Late Effect codes can be used at any time after the acute injury. Examples of these are:

- 906.3: Late effect of contusion
- 908.0: Late effect of internal injury to chest

Examples of Late Effects With the Cause

Cause	Late Effect
Fracture	Malunion
Cardiovascular accident	Hemiplegia
Third-degree burn	Deep scarring
Polio	Contractures
Laceration	Keloids
Breast implants	Ruptured implant

Truncated Diagnosis Code

A truncated diagnosis code is one that does not have the required 4th or 5th digit.

There are fewer than 100 codes that are three-digit codes; all others require additional digits for billing. It is the responsibility of the provider to assign the diagnosis codes.

(Continued text on following page)

Example: Abdominal Pain 789.$\underline{0}$ (requires a 5th digit)

0 Unspecified site	5 Periumbilical
1 Right upper quadrant	6 Epigastric
2 Left upper quadrant	7 Generalized
3 Right lower quadrant	8 Other specified site
4 Left lower quadrant	

Multiple Diagnosis Codes

■ All diagnosis codes must be prioritized in order of significance and linked to the appropriate procedure or service

■ When coding both surgical and medical problems for the same patient, list the surgical problem first. When the severity of the medical problem supersedes the importance of the surgical problem, then list the medical problem first.

■ A maximum of four diagnosis codes can be submitted per claim.

Nonspecific/Unspecified Codes

Codes that are referred to as nonspecific or unspecified are not the most specific codes possible for the reporting of the diagnosis or condition. In Volume 1, these codes are listed as NOS (not otherwise specified); in Volume 2, they are listed as NEC (not elsewhere classified).
Examples of these codes are:

■ 420.90: Acute pericarditis, unspecified NOS

■ 682.9: Cellulitis, NOS

■ 599.0: Infection, genitourinary tract NEC

Signs and Symptoms Codes

When a definitive diagnosis code is not available, use a sign or symptom code.

Example: Suspected pneumonia, but not sure until x-ray. Diagnoses used for this visit would be the symptoms of the patient.

- Wheeze
- Shortness of breath
- Fever
- Cough

Example: Possible fracture of wrist, but not sure until x-ray. Diagnoses used for this visit would be the symptoms of the patient.

- Swelling
- Pain in wrist

ICD-9-CM Guidelines for Coding and Reporting

- Identify each service, procedure, or supply with a diagnosis code
- Chronic diseases should be reported, if appropriate
- Always use the code with the highest degree of specificity; add 4th and 5th digits when appropriate
- Properly link all diagnosis codes to the CPT code
- Do not code using "rule-out," "suspected," "probable," "questionable," etc.
- Use signs and symptoms when a definitive diagnosis code is not available.
- Code the primary diagnosis first, followed by the secondary, tertiary, and so on
- Do not use a diagnosis code that is no longer applicable
- For surgical procedures, code the diagnosis applicable to the procedure; if at the time the claim is filed, the postoperative diagnosis is different from the preoperative diagnosis, use the postoperative diagnosis for billing

Principal Versus Primary Diagnosis Code

- **Principal diagnosis:** reported on inpatient hospital claims (facility, Part A Medicare); reported on UB-92 form; the principal diagnosis is the condition determined *after the study* that resulted in the patient's admission to the hospital
- **Primary diagnosis:** reported by the physician (professional, Part B Medicare); reported on HCFA 1500 claim form; the primary diagnosis is the most significant condition for which services and/or procedures were provided

Hypertension/Hypertensive Table

The hypertension table is a complete listing of hypertension codes and conditions associated with hypertension. The table consists of three columns:

1. Malignant
2. Benign
3. Unspecified

Malignant hypertension is a form with vascular damage and a diastolic blood pressure reading of 130 mm Hg or greater.
Benign hypertension is a form of mild or controlled hypertension with no damage to the patient's vascular system or organs.
Unspecified hypertension is reflected by no notation of benign or malignant status in the patient's medical record.

Neoplasm Table

Neoplasms are new growths in which cell reproduction is out of control. It is important to know whether the tumor is malignant or benign. Malignant is when the growth is cancerous, invasive, or capable of spreading to other parts of the body. Benign is when the growth is noncancerous, nonmalignant, or noninvasive.

The Neoplasm Table is arranged by anatomical site and contains four classifications:

Type of Neoplasm	Description
Malignant ■ Primary ■ Secondary ■ Ca in Situ	■ **Primary malignant** growth is the original tumor site. All malignant tumors are considered primary unless otherwise noted as metastatic or secondary. ■ **Secondary malignant** growth is where the tumor has metastasized (spread) to a secondary site, either adjacent to the primary site or to a remote region of the body. ■ **Ca in situ** is a malignant tumor that is localized, circumscribed, encapsulated, and noninvasive (has not spread to other tissues or organs).
Benign	A **benign** growth is a noninvasive, nonspreading, nonmalignant tumor
Uncertain behavior	**Uncertain behavior** is a type of growth by which it is not possible to predict subsequent morphology or behavior from the submitted specimen. In order to assign a code from this column, the pathology report must specifically indicate the "uncertain behavior" of the neoplasm.
Unspecified nature	**Unspecified nature** is a type of growth where a neoplasm is identified, but there is no further indication of the histology or nature of the tumor reflected in the documented diagnosis. Assign a code from this column when the neoplasm was destroyed or removed and a tissue biopsy was performed and results are pending.

Hint: If the statement does not classify the neoplasm, refer to the Index to Diseases entry for the condition documented instead of the table. That entry will contain a code that can be cross-checked in the table.

Primary Malignancies

Primary malignancies are coded if the note in the medical record states:

- Metastatic *from* a site
- Spread *from* a site
- *Primary* neoplasm of a site
- A malignancy for which no specific classification is documented
- A *recurrent* tumor

Example: Carcinoma of the **cervical lymph nodes**; metastatic from the **breast**
Primary: breast
Secondary: cervical lymph nodes

Secondary Malignancies

Secondary malignancies are metastatic and indicate that a primary cancer spread to another part of the body.
Example: Metastatic carcinoma from breast to lung
Assign two codes:

1) Primary malignant neoplasm of the breast: 174.9
2) Secondary neoplasm of the lung: 197.0

The following lists secondary sites for malignancies:

1. Bone
2. Brain
3. Diaphragm
4. Heart
5. Liver
6. Lymph nodes
7. Mediastinum
8. Meninges
9. Peritoneum
10. Pleura
11. Retroperitoneum
12. Spinal cord

Re-excision

A re-excision occurs when a pathologist recommends that the surgeon perform a second excision to widen the margins of the original tumor site. The pathology report may not specify a malignancy at this time, but the patient is still under treatment for the original neoplasm.

M Codes

M codes are morphology of neoplasm codes. They are used to report the type of neoplasm. They are used by the hospital to report neoplasms to the cancer registry.
Examples of these codes are:

■ M8041/3: Small cell carcinoma NOS
■ M8000/0: Neoplasm, benign

Table of Drugs and Chemicals

The table lists drugs and chemicals that have caused a poisoning or adverse effect. It is divided into six External Cause codes:

	External Cause	Description	Codes
1	Poisoning	These codes are assigned according to the classification of the drug or chemical involved in the poisoning	960–989
2	Accident	These codes are used for accidental overdosing, wrong substance given or taken, drug inadvertently taken, or accidents in the use of drugs and chemical substances during a medical or surgical procedure	E850–E869

(Continued text on following page)

	External Cause	Description	Codes
3	Therapeutic use	These codes are used for the external effect caused by correct substance properly administered in therapeutic or prophylactic dosages	E930–E952
4	Suicide attempt	These codes are used to report self-inflicted poisonings	E950–E952
5	Assault	These codes represent a poisoning inflicted by another person who intended to kill or injure the patient	E961–E962
6	Undetermined	These codes are used if the record does not state whether the poisoning was intentional or accidental	E980–E982

Fracture Coding

When coding fractures, if the note does not state if the fracture is open or closed, assume that it is closed, and code it appropriately. When dealing with multiple injuries, list them in descending order of severity.

Types of Fractures

Types of Closed Fractures	Description
Comminuted	Has more than two fragments of bone that are broken off; it is unstable and contains many bone fragments and tissue damage
Linear	The fracture runs along the length of the bone

Types of Closed Fractures	Description
Spiral	The bone is broken as a result of a twisting motion; this fracture is sometimes confused with an oblique fracture
Depressed	Skull fracture with the bone forced inwards
Simple	Fracture does not break the skin and has little, if any, tissue damage
Impact/ Compression	The vertebral column is compressed and then breaks under the pressure
Complex	Fracture that severely damages the soft tissue around the fracture site
Stress	A fracture caused by repeated stress to the bone
Double	Multiple fractures of the same bone occurring at the same time
Greenstick	Bendlike fracture found mostly in children; the bone is not broken through
Impacted	The bones are broken and the ends are smashed together in a head-on fashion
Fragmented	A fracture in which the trauma leaves many broken bones inside the patient
Oblique	Facture forms an oblique break in the bone; very rare
Fissure	Also known as a hairline fracture; minimal trauma to the bone and tissues; it is an incomplete fracture, as it is not all the way through the bone
Closed	There is a fracture with no broken skin
Infected	A fracture in which the area has become infected
Compound/Open	A fracture that breaks the skin
Pathological	Fracture is caused by some type of disease process

Modifiers/HCPCS Coding
(National Codes) Level II

Modifiers are two- to five-digit numeric or alphanumeric characters that can be reported with CPT codes. They provide additional information regarding the code to which they are attached. These codes indicate that the CPT code has been altered in some way, but the basic code is the same.

When to use a modifier:

1. Only part of a service or procedure is performed
2. A service or procedure has been reduced
3. A service or procedure has been increased
4. Unusual circumstances surround the service or procedure
5. The service or procedure was performed multiple times
6. The procedure was bilateral
7. The procedure can be reported either as a technical or professional service
8. An adjunctive service was performed
9. The service or procedure was performed by more than one physician
10. The service or procedure was performed in more than one location
11. For anesthesia: when the physical status of the patient needs to be reported for the administration of anesthesia

Types of Modifiers

Abbreviation	Modifier Use With:	Code Range
E&M	Evaluation and Management Codes	99201–99499
A	Anesthesia Codes	00100–01999
S	Surgery Codes	10021–69990
R	Radiology Codes	70010–79999
P	Pathology and Laboratory Codes	80048–89356
M	Medicine Codes	90281–99602

Some modifiers are used as informational only and do not affect reimbursement of the claim. These informational modifiers **can affect** whether the claim will be paid or denied. Others, however, can affect reimbursement.

*Current Procedural Terminology © 2006 American Medical Association, All Rights Reserved.

Evaluation and Management (E&M) Code Modifiers

The modifiers used with E&M codes are -21, -24, -25, -32, -52, -57.

Modifier -21	Description	Effect on Payment	Accepted by Medicare
	Prolonged E&M Service	No	Yes

Used to identify face-to-face time with a patient that is prolonged or greater than normal.

Modifier -24	Description	Effect on Payment	Accepted by Medicare
	Unrelated E&M service by the same physician during postop period	Yes; failure to use modifier may cause claim denials	Yes

Indicate that the E&M service performed during a postoperative period was not related to the procedure performed.

Modifier -25	Description	Effect on Payment	Accepted by Medicare
	Significant separately identifiable E&M service by the same physician on the same day of a procedure	Yes, failure to use modifier may cause claim denials	Yes

When necessary to perform a separate service, above and beyond the procedure performed.

*Current Procedural Terminology © 2006 American Medical Association, All Rights Reserved.

MOD/
HCPCS

Modifier -32	Description	Effect on Payment	Accepted by Medicare
	Mandated service	No	Yes

When necessary to provide an E&M service at the request of a third-party carrier, government, or peer review organization.

Modifier -52	Description	Effect on Payment	Accepted by Medicare
	Reduced service	Yes	Yes

When necessary to report a reduced E&M service when a complete service is not performed.

Modifier -57	Description	Effect on Payment	Accepted by Medicare
	Decision for surgery	Yes	Yes

It may be necessary to report an E&M service that resulted in a decision to perform surgery. This service would be performed the day prior to and/or on the day of the surgery. CPT codes used with the -57 modifier are 92002–92014 and 99201–99499.

Anesthesia Modifiers

The modifiers used with anesthesia codes are -22, -23, -32, -47, -51, -53, -59.

Modifier -22	Description	Effect on Payment	Accepted by Medicare
	Unusual procedural service	Yes	Yes

When necessary to report a procedure that is greater than that normally required.

Modifier -23	Description	Effect on Payment	Accepted by Medicare
	Unusual anesthesia	Yes	Yes

When necessary to report a procedure that usually requires no anesthesia, local anesthesia, or general anesthesia.

Modifier -32	Description	Effect on Payment	Accepted by Medicare
	Mandated service	No	Yes

When necessary to provide an E&M service at the request of a third-party carrier, government, or peer review organization.

Modifier -47	Description	Effect on Payment	Accepted by Medicare
	Anesthesia by surgeon	No	No

Used when regional or general anesthesia is provided by the surgeon without an anesthesiologist or CRNA involvement.

Modifier -51	Description	Effect on Payment	Accepted by Medicare
	Multiple procedures	Yes	Yes

Used when multiple procedures, other than E&M services, are performed at the same session by the same provider.

Modifier -53	Description	Effect on Payment	Accepted by Medicare
	Discontinued procedure	Yes	Yes

Used when procedures are terminated after they are started or after anesthesia is started due to extenuating circumstances or a threat to the patient's health.

*Current Procedural Terminology © 2006 American Medical Association, All Rights Reserved.

MOD/
HCPCS

Modifier -59	Description	Effect on Payment	Accepted by Medicare
	Distinct procedural service	Yes	Yes

Used when procedures not usually performed together are performed, distinct, and medically necessary.

Surgery Modifiers

The modifiers used with surgery codes are -22, -26, -32, -47, -50, -51, -52, -53, -54, -55, -56, -58, -59, -62, -66, -76, -77, -78, -79, -80, -81, -82, -99.

Modifier -22	Description	Effect on Payment	Accepted by Medicare
	Unusual procedural service	Yes	Yes

When necessary to report a procedure that is greater than that normally required.

Modifier -26	Description	Effect on Payment	Accepted by Medicare
	Professional component	Yes	Yes

When necessary to report only a physician's interpretation of a test.

Modifier -32	Description	Effect on Payment	Accepted by Medicare
	Mandated service	No	Yes

When necessary to provide an E&M service at the request of a third-party carrier, government, or peer review organization.

Modifier -47	Description	Effect on Payment	Accepted by Medicare
	Anesthesia by surgeon	No	No

Used when regional or general anesthesia is provided by the surgeon without an anesthesiologist or CRNA involvement.

Modifier -50	Description	Effect on Payment	Accepted by Medicare
	Bilateral procedure	Yes	Yes

Used to report bilateral procedures performed at the same operative session.

Modifier -51	Description	Effect on Payment	Accepted by Medicare
	Multiple procedures	Yes	Yes

Used when multiple procedures, other than E&M services, are performed at the same session by the same provider.

Modifier -52	Description	Effect on Payment	Accepted by Medicare
	Reduced service	Yes	Yes

Used when necessary to report a reduced E&M service when a complete service is not performed.

Modifier -53	Description	Effect on Payment	Accepted by Medicare
	Discontinued procedure	Yes	Yes

MOD/ HCPCS

Used when procedures are terminated after they are started or after anesthesia is started due to extenuating circumstances or a threat to the patient's health.

Modifier -54	Description	Effect on Payment	Accepted by Medicare
	Surgical care only	Yes	Yes

Used to report a procedure when a physician performs the procedure and another physician performs the postoperative care.

Modifier -55	Description	Effect on Payment	Accepted by Medicare
	Postoperative care only	Yes	Yes

Used to report a procedure when a physician performs the postoperative care only and another surgeon performs the procedure.

Modifier -56	Description	Effect on Payment	Accepted by Medicare
	Postoperative care only	Yes	No

Used to report when a physician performs the preoperative care and another physician performs the procedure.

Modifier -58	Description	Effect on Payment	Accepted by Medicare
	Staged or related procedure or service by the same physician during postoperative period.	Yes	Yes

Used to report when the same physician performs a staged or related procedure during the postoperative period.

Modifier -59	Description	Effect on Payment	Accepted by Medicare
	Distinct procedural service	Yes	Yes

Used when procedures not usually performed together are performed, are distinct, and are medically necessary.

Modifier -62	Description	Effect on Payment	Accepted by Medicare
	Two surgeons	Yes	Yes

Used when two surgeons work together as primary surgeons if the procedure is so complex that it requires two surgeons to manage. Each surgeon is of a different specialty. CPT codes that can be used with the -62 modifier are 10040–69979, 70010–79999, and 90281–99199

Modifier -66	Description	Effect on Payment	Accepted by Medicare
	Surgical team	Yes	Yes

Used when procedures that are extremely complex are performed under a surgical team concept.

Modifier -76	Description	Effect on Payment	Accepted by Medicare
	Repeat procedure by same physician	Yes	Yes

Used when the same physician repeats the exact same service.

Modifier -77	Description	Effect on Payment	Accepted by Medicare
	Repeat procedure by another physician	Yes	Yes

Used when a procedure is repeated by a different physician at a separate time on the same day.

*Current Procedural Terminology © 2006 American Medical Association, All Rights Reserved.

MOD/ HCPCS

Modifier -78	Description	Effect on Payment	Accepted by Medicare
	Return to operating room for a related procedure during postop	Yes	Yes

Used when a patient needs to return to the operating room to treat complications of the original surgery.

Modifier -79	Description	Effect on Payment	Accepted by Medicare
	Unrelated procedure or service by the same physician during postop	Yes	Yes

Used when an unrelated procedure is performed by the same physician during the postoperative period of the original procedure.

Modifier -80	Description	Effect on Payment	Accepted by Medicare
	Assistant surgeon	Yes	Yes

Used to identify the services of an assistant surgeon necessary for a procedure.

Modifier -81	Description	Effect on Payment	Accepted by Medicare
	Minimum assistant surgeon	Yes	Yes

Used when the services of additional surgeons (second or third assistant) are required for a procedure.

Modifier -82	Description	Effect on Payment	Accepted by Medicare
	Assistant surgeon, when a qualified resident is unavailable	Yes	Yes

Used when a surgical assist is necessary for a procedure, but there is no resident available.

Modifier -99	Description	Effect on Payment	Accepted by Medicare
	Multiple modifiers	No	Yes

Used to report that there are multiple modifiers being used for this claim.

Radiology Modifiers

The modifiers used with radiology codes are -22, -26, -32, -50, -51, -52, -53, -58, -59, -62, -76, -77, -78, -79, -80, -99.

Modifier -22	Description	Effect on Payment	Accepted by Medicare
	Unusual procedural service	Yes	Yes

Used when necessary to report a procedure that is greater than that normally required.

Modifier -26	Description	Effect on Payment	Accepted by Medicare
	Professional component	Yes	Yes

Used when necessary to report only a physician's interpretation of a test.

*Current Procedural Terminology © 2006 American Medical Association, All Rights Reserved.

MOD/ HCPCS

Modifier -32	Description	Effect on Payment	Accepted by Medicare
	Mandated service	No	Yes

Used when necessary to provide an E&M service at the request of a third-party carrier, government, or peer review organization.

Modifier -50	Description	Effect on Payment	Accepted by Medicare
	Bilateral procedure	Yes	Yes

Used to report bilateral procedures performed at the same operative session.

Modifier -51	Description	Effect on Payment	Accepted by Medicare
	Multiple procedures	Yes	Yes

Used when multiple procedures, other than E&M services, are performed at the same session by the same provider.

Modifier -52	Description	Effect on Payment	Accepted by Medicare
	Reduced service	Yes	Yes

When necessary to report a reduced E&M service when a complete service is not performed.

Modifier -53	Description	Effect on Payment	Accepted by Medicare
	Discontinued procedure	Yes	Yes

Used when procedures are terminated after they are started or after anesthesia is started due to extenuating circumstances or a threat to the patient's health.

Modifier -58	Description	Effect on Payment	Accepted by Medicare
	Staged or related procedure or service by the same physician during postop	Yes	Yes

Used to report when the same physician performs a staged or related procedure during the postoperative period.

Modifier -59	Description	Effect on Payment	Accepted by Medicare
	Distinct procedural service	Yes	Yes

Used when procedures not usually performed together are performed, are distinct, and are medically necessary.

Modifier -62	Description	Effect on Payment	Accepted by Medicare
	Two surgeons	Yes	Yes

Used when two surgeons work together as primary surgeons if the procedure is so complex that it requires two surgeons to manage.

Modifier -76	Description	Effect on Payment	Accepted by Medicare
	Repeat procedure by same physician	Yes	Yes

Used when the same physician repeats the exact same service.

*Current Procedural Terminology © 2006 American Medical Association, All Rights Reserved.

Modifier -77	Description	Effect on Payment	Accepted by Medicare
	Repeat procedure by another physician	Yes	Yes

Used when a procedure is repeated by a different physician at a separate time on the same day.

Modifier -78	Description	Effect on Payment	Accepted by Medicare
	Return to operating room for a related procedure during the post-operative period	Yes	Yes

Used when a patient needs to return to the operating room to treat complications of the original surgery.

Modifier -79	Description	Effect on Payment	Accepted by Medicare
	Unrelated procedure or service by the same physician during the post-operative period	Yes	Yes

Used when an unrelated procedure is performed by the same physician during the postoperative period of the original procedure.

Modifier -80	Description	Effect on Payment	Accepted by Medicare
	Assistant surgeon	Yes	Yes

Used to identify the services of an assistant surgeon necessary for a procedure.

Modifier -99	Description	Effect on Payment	Accepted by Medicare
	Multiple modifiers	No	Yes

Used to report that there are multiple modifiers being used for this claim.

Pathology and Laboratory Modifiers

The modifiers used with pathology and laboratory codes are -22, -26, -32, -52, -53, -59, -90, -91.

Modifier -22	Description	Effect on Payment	Accepted by Medicare
	Unusual procedural service	Yes	Yes

When necessary to report a procedure that is greater than that normally required.

Modifier -26	Description	Effect on Payment	Accepted by Medicare
	Professional component	Yes	Yes

When necessary to report only a physician's interpretation of a test.

Modifier -32	Description	Effect on Payment	Accepted by Medicare
	Mandated service	No	Yes

When necessary to provide an E&M service at the request of a third-party carrier, government, or peer review organization.

*Current Procedural Terminology © 2006 American Medical Association, All Rights Reserved.

MOD/
HCPCS

Modifier -52	Description	Effect on Payment	Accepted by Medicare
	Reduced service	Yes	Yes

Used when necessary to report a reduced E&M service when a complete service is not performed.

Modifier -53	Description	Effect on Payment	Accepted by Medicare
	Discontinued procedure	Yes	Yes

Used when procedures are terminated after they are started or after anesthesia is started due to extenuating circumstances or a threat to the patient's health.

Modifier -59	Description	Effect on Payment	Accepted by Medicare
	Distinct procedural service	Yes	Yes

Used when procedures not usually performed together are performed, are distinct, and are medically necessary.

Modifier -90	Description	Effect on Payment	Accepted by Medicare
	Reference (outside) laboratory	No	No

Used when laboratory tests are performed by a laboratory other than that of the reporting physician.

Modifier -91	Description	Effect on Payment	Accepted by Medicare
	Repeat clinical diagnostic laboratory test	Yes	Yes

Used when laboratory tests are performed on specimens from the same patient source more than one time on the same day.

Medicine Modifiers

The modifiers used with pathology and laboratory codes are -22, -26, -32, -50, -51, -52, -53, -55, -56, 58, -59, -76, -77, -78, -79, -99.

Modifier -22	Description	Effect on Payment	Accepted by Medicare
	Unusual procedural service	Yes	Yes

Used when necessary to report a procedure that is greater than that normally required.

Modifier -26	Description	Effect on Payment	Accepted by Medicare
	Professional component	Yes	Yes

Used when necessary to report only a physician's interpretation of a test.

Modifier -32	Description	Effect on Payment	Accepted by Medicare
	Mandated service	No	Yes

Used when necessary to provide an E&M service at the request of a third-party carrier, government, or peer review organization.

Modifier -50	Description	Effect on Payment	Accepted by Medicare
	Bilateral procedure	Yes	Yes

Used to report bilateral procedures performed at the same operative session.

---

*Current Procedural Terminology © 2006 American Medical Association, All Rights Reserved.

Modifier -51	Description	Effect on Payment	Accepted by Medicare
	Multiple procedures	Yes	Yes

Used when multiple procedures, other than E&M services, are performed at the same session by the same provider.

Modifier -52	Description	Effect on Payment	Accepted by Medicare
	Reduced service	Yes	Yes

Used when necessary to report a reduced E&M service when a complete service is not performed.

Modifier -53	Description	Effect on Payment	Accepted by Medicare
	Discontinued procedure	Yes	Yes

Used when procedures are terminated after they are started or after anesthesia is started due to extenuating circumstances or a threat to the patient's health.

Modifier -55	Description	Effect on Payment	Accepted by Medicare
	Postoperative care only	Yes	Yes

Used to report a procedure when a physician performs the postoperative care only and another surgeon performs the procedure.

Modifier -56	Description	Effect on Payment	Accepted by Medicare
	Preoperative care only	Yes	No

Used to report when one physician performs the preoperative care and another physician performs the procedure.

Modifier -58	Description	Effect on Payment	Accepted by Medicare
	Staged or related procedure or service by the same physician during postop	Yes	Yes

Used to report when the same physician performs a staged or related procedure during the postoperative period.

Modifier -59	Description	Effect on Payment	Accepted by Medicare
	Distinct procedural service	Yes	Yes

Used when procedures not usually performed together are performed, are distinct, and are medically necessary.

Modifier -76	Description	Effect on Payment	Accepted by Medicare
	Repeat procedure by same physician	Yes	Yes

Used when the same physician repeats the exact same service.

Modifier -77	Description	Effect on Payment	Accepted by Medicare
	Repeat procedure by another physician	Yes	Yes

Used when a procedure is repeated by a different physician at a separate time on the same day.

Modifier -78	Description	Effect on Payment	Accepted by Medicare
	Return to operating room for a related procedure during the postoperative period	Yes	Yes

*Current Procedural Terminology © 2006 American Medical Association, All Rights Reserved.

MOD/
HCPCS

Used when a patient needs to return to the operating room to treat complications of the original surgery.

Modifier -79	Description	Effect on Payment	Accepted by Medicare
	Unrelated procedure or service by the same physician during the postoperative period	Yes	Yes

Used when an unrelated procedure is performed by the same physician during the postoperative period of the original procedure.

Modifier -99	Description	Effect on Payment	Accepted by Medicare
	Multiple modifiers	No	Yes

Used to report that there are multiple modifiers being used for this claim.

Ambulatory Surgery Center (ASC)/ Hospital Outpatient Modifiers

The modifiers used in ASC billing are -25, -27, -50, -52, -58, -59, -73, -74, -76, -77, -78, -79, -91.

Modifier -25	Description	Effect on Payment	Accepted by Medicare
	Significant, separately identifiable E&M service by the same physician on the same day of a procedure	Yes; failure to use modifier may cause claim denials	Yes

When necessary to perform a separate service above and beyond the procedure performed. Should also be used with Preventive Medicine services when patient also presents with a complaint that requires further treatment or testing. CPT codes that can be used with the -25 modifier are 92002–92014 and 99201–99499.

Modifier -27	Description	Effect on Payment	Accepted by Medicare
	Multiple outpatient hospital E&M services on the same date	Yes	Yes

Used for facility billing only. It is used to report the utilization of hospital resources related to separate and distinct E&M services performed in multiple outpatient hospital settings on the same date.

Modifier -50	Description	Effect on Payment	Accepted by Medicare
	Bilateral procedure	Yes	Yes

Used to report bilateral procedures performed at the same operative session. Add the -50 modifier to the second procedure. Do not use with codes that are performed bilaterally.

Modifier -52	Description	Effect on Payment	Accepted by Medicare
	Reduced service	Yes	Yes

Used when necessary to report a reduced E&M service when a complete service is not performed.

Modifier -58	Description	Effect on Payment	Accepted by Medicare
	Staged or related procedure or service by the same physician during the post-operative period.	Yes	Yes

*Current Procedural Terminology © 2006 American Medical Association, All Rights Reserved.

Used when the same physician performs a staged or related procedure during the postoperative period.

Modifier -59	Description	Effect on Payment	Accepted by Medicare
	Distinct procedural service	Yes	Yes

Used when procedures not usually performed together are performed, are distinct, and are medically necessary.

Modifier -73	Description	Effect on Payment	Accepted by Medicare
	Discontinued outpatient hospital/ ambulatory surgery center (ASC) prior to the administration of anesthesia	Yes	Yes

Used when there are extenuating circumstances that may threaten the well-being of the patient and cause the physician to cancel or postpone the procedure.

Modifier -74	Description	Effect on Payment	Accepted by Medicare
	Discontinued outpatient hospital/ambulatory surgery center (ASC) prior to the adminis-tration of anesthesia	Yes	Yes

Used when there are extenuating circumstances that may threaten the well-being of the patient and cause the physician to cancel or postpone the procedure after administration of anesthesia.

Modifier -76	Description	Effect on Payment	Accepted by Medicare
	Repeat procedure by same physician	Yes	Yes

Used when the same physician repeats the exact same service.

Modifier -77	Description	Effect on Payment	Accepted by Medicare
	Repeat procedure by another physician	Yes	Yes

Used when a procedure is repeated by a different physician at a separate time on the same day.

Modifier -78	Description	Effect on Payment	Accepted by Medicare
	Return to operating room for a related procedure during the postoperative period	Yes	Yes

Used when a patient needs to return to the operating room to treat complications of the original surgery.

Modifier -79	Description	Effect on Payment	Accepted by Medicare
	Unrelated procedure or service by the same physician during the postoperative period	Yes	Yes

Used when an unrelated procedure is performed by the same physician during the postoperative period of the original procedure.

---

*Current Procedural Terminology © 2006 American Medical Association, All Rights Reserved.

MOD/
HCPCS

Modifier -91	Description	Effect on Payment	Accepted by Medicare
	Repeat clinical diagnostic laboratory test	Yes	Yes

Used when laboratory tests are performed on specimens from the same patient source more than one time on the same day.

Teaching Physician Modifiers

The following two modifiers are used in a teaching physician setting when a resident is involved in the service. These modifiers have no effect on payment and are used only to track the medical education funds.

Modifier -GC	Description	Effect on Payment	Accepted by Medicare
	The service has been performed in part by a resident under the direction of a teaching physician	No	Yes

Modifier -GE	Description	Effect on Payment	Accepted by Medicare
	The service has been performed by a resident without the presence of a teaching physician	No	Yes

This modifier is used when services are provided under the primary care exemption.

HCPCS Coding (National Codes) Level II

The Healthcare Common Procedure Coding System (HCPCS) was designed to enable providers to report such things as services, procedures, and supplies. These codes are used to report nonphysician services, supplies, and durable medical equipment (DME). These codes are alphanumeric: one letter (A through V, no S) with four numbers. An updated version of this book is released in the fall of each year. This book should be purchased each year, as there are many changes that may cause delays and denials in claims should the provider not be aware of them. There is no grace period for these codes. All codes must be implemented on January 1 of each year. There are two levels of HCPCS codes:

1. Level I: CPT book – see Tabs 2-5
2. Level II: national codes found in an HCPCS code book – this tab

General Rule

There are instances when both a CPT and HCPCS code exists for the same service or procedure. When this occurs and both the CPT code and HCPCS code have identical descriptions, the CPT code is used. If the descriptions are not identical, use the HCPCS code. There are times when the CPT code listed is not as specific as the HCPCS code.

Steps for Using the HCPCS Book

1. Determine the service, procedure, or supply received
2. Look up the term in the index at the beginning of the HCPCS book
3. Assign a provisional code
4. Locate the provisional code in the appropriate section of the HCPCS book
5. Check for any colors, symbols, notes, etc.
6. Review the appendices for any guidelines that may be relevant
7. Attach a modifier, if applicable
8. Enter the HCPCS code into the computer or on the claim form

*Current Procedural Terminology © 2006 American Medical Association, All Rights Reserved.

Categories of the HCPCS Level II Book

Main Book

1. Index
2. Transportation Services including Ambulance
3. Medical Surgical Supplies
4. Administrative, Miscellaneous, and Investigational
5. Enteral and Parenteral Therapy
6. Outpatient PPS
7. Dental Procedures
8. Durable Medical Equipment (DME)
9. Procedures/Professional Services (temporary)
10. Alcohol and Drug Abuse Treatment Services
11. Drug Administered Other Than Oral Method
12. Chemotherapy Drugs
13. Temporary Codes
14. Orthotic Procedures
15. Prosthetic Procedures
16. Medical Services
17. Pathology and Laboratory Services
18. Q Codes (temporary)
19. Diagnostic Radiology Services
20. Temporary National Codes (Non-Medicare)
21. National T Codes
22. Vision Services
23. Hearing Services

Appendices

24. Modifiers
25. Abbreviations
26. Table of Drugs
27. National Coverage Determinations Manual
28. National Average Payment

Below are examples by section of commonly used HCPCS codes:

To report these codes, use CMS Form 1491

Transportation Services Including Ambulance (Codes A0021–A0999)

Code	Description
A0100	Nonemergency transportation; taxi
A0424	Extra ambulance attendant, ground or air
A0426	Ambulance service, advanced life support, nonemergency, level 1 (ALS)
A0428	Ambulance service, basic life support, nonemergency

Ambulance origin and destination modifiers are used with transportation service codes. Assign the origin modifier first and place the destination modifier second in boxes 12 and 13 of the form.

Modifier	Description
D	Diagnostic or therapeutic site other than P or H
E	Residential, domiciliary, custodial facility (nursing home, not skilled nursing facility)
G	Hospital-based dialysis facility
H	Hospital
I	Site of transfer (helicopter pad, etc.) between types of ambulance
J	Nonhospital-based dialysis facility
N	Skilled nursing facility (SNF)
P	Physician's office
R	Residence
S	Scene of accident or acute event (stadium, prison, school)
X	Intermediate stop at physician's office en route to the hospital

Medical Surgical Supplies (Codes A4206–A7527)

Code	Description
A4211	Supplies for self-administered injections
A4250	Urine test strips (100)
A4561	Pessary, rubber, any type
A4570	Splint

Administrative, Miscellaneous, and Investigational (Codes A9150–A9999)

Code	Description
A9150	Nonprescription drug
A9280	Alert, alarm device
A9700	Supply of injectable contrast material for use in echocardiography, per study
A9901	DME delivery, set up and/or dispensing service component of another HCPCS code

Enteral and Parenteral Therapy (Codes B4034–B9999)

Code	Description
B4034	Enteral feeding supply kit; syringe, per day
B4081	Nasogastric tubing with stylet
B4100	Food thickener
B4103	Enteral formula, for pediatric, used to replace fluids and electrolytes

Outpatient PPS (Codes C1079–C9722)	
Code	Description
C1785	Pacemaker, dual chamber, rate-responsive
C1788	Port, indwelling (implantable)
C8906	Magnetic resonance imaging with contrast, breast; bilateral
C9405	Supply of radiopharmaceutical therapeutic diagnostic agent I-131 sodium iodide capsule, per MCI, brand name

Dental Procedures (Codes D0120–D9999)	
Code	Description
D0120	Periodic oral examination
D0170	Reevaluation—limited, problem-focused (established patient; not post-op)
D0330	Panoramic film
D2932	Prefabricated resin crown

Durable Medical Equipment (DME) (Codes E0100–E8002)	
Code	Description
E0140	Walker, folding (pick-up), adjustable or adjustable height
E0720	TENS, two lead, localized stimulation
E0860	Traction equipment, over door
E1240	Lightweight wheelchair; detachable arms, desk or full-length, swing-away, elevating leg rests

MOD/
HCPCS

Procedures/Professional Services (temporary) (Codes G0008–G9037)

Code	Description
G0117	Glaucoma screening for high-risk patients furnished by an optometrist or ophthalmologist
G0121	Colorectal cancer screening; colonoscopy on individual not meeting criteria for high risk
G0226	PET imaging whole body; diagnosis; esophageal cancer
G0359	Chemotherapy administration, intravenous infusion technique; up to 1 hour, single or initial substance/drug

Alcohol and Drug Abuse Treatment Services (Codes H0001–H2037)

Code	Description
H0001	Alcohol and/or drug assessment
H1000	Prenatal care, at-risk assessment
H2011	Crisis intervention service, per 15 minutes
H2035	Alcohol and/or drug treatment program, per hour

Drug Administered Other Than Oral Method (Codes J0120–J8999)

Code	Description
J0170	Injection, adrenalin, epinephrine, up to 1 mL ampule
J1040	Injection, methylprednisolone acetate, 80 mg
J1642	Injection, heparin sodium, (heparin lock flush), per 10 units
J2175	Injection meperidine HCl, per 100 mg

Chemotherapy Drugs (Codes J9000–J9999)

Code	Description
J9000	Doxorubicin HCl, 10 mg (Adriamycin)
J9062	Cisplatin, 50 mg (Platinol AQ)
J9080	Cyclophosphamide, 200 mg (Cytoxin, Neosar)
J9218	Luprolide acetate, per 1 mg (Lupron)

Temporary Codes (Codes K0001–K0669)

Code	Description
K0010	Standard-weight frame motorized/power wheelchair
K0416	Prescription antiemetic drug, rectal, per 1 mg, for use in conjunction with oral anticancer drug
K0552	Supplies for external drug infusion pump, syringe-type cartridge, sterile, each
K0620	Tubular elastic dressing, any width, per linear yard

Orthotic Procedures (Codes L0100–L4398)

Code	Description
L0210	Thoracic rib belt
L3201	Orthopedic shoe, Oxford with supinator or pronator, infant
L3215	Orthopedic footwear, woman's shoes
L3480	Heel pad and depression for spur

Prosthetic Procedures (Codes L5000–L9900)	
Code	Description
L5000	Partial foot, shoe inset with longitudinal arch, toe filler
L5700	Replacement, socket, below knee, molded to patient model
L8600	Implantable breast prosthesis, silicone or equal
L8614	Cochlear device system

Medical Services (Codes M0064–M0301)	
Code	Description
M0064	Brief office visit for the sole purpose of monitoring or changing drug prescription used in the treatment of mental psychoneurotic and personality disorders
M0076	Prolotherapy
M0300	IV chelation therapy
M0301	Fabric wrapping of abdominal aneurysm

Pathology and Laboratory Services (Codes P2028–P9615)	
Code	Description
P3000	Screening Pap smear, cervical or vaginal, up to three smears, by technician under physician supervision
P7001	Culture, bacterial, urine, quantitative, sensitivity study
P9010	Whole blood for transfusion, per unit
P9612	Catheterization for collection of specimen(s), single patient

Q Codes (temporary) ¡Codes Q0035–Q4077)

Code	Description
Q0081	Infusion therapy, using other than chemotherapeutic drugs, per visit
Q0091	Screening Pap smear, obtaining, preparing, and conveyance of cervical or vaginal smear to laboratory
Q0136	Injection, epoetin alpha, for non-ESRD use, per 1000 units
Q3031	Collagen skin test

Diagnostic Radiology Services (Codes R0070–R0076)

Code	Description
R0070	Transportation of portable x-ray equipment and personnel to home or nursing home, per trip to facility or location, one patient seen
R0075	Transportation of portable x-ray equipment and personnel to home or nursing home, per trip to facility or location, more than one patient seen
R0076	Transportation of portable EKG to facility or location, one patient

Temporary National Codes (Non-Medicare) (Codes S0012–S9999)

Code	Description
S0390	Routine foot care; removal and/or trimming of corns, calluses and/or nails and preventive maintenance in specific medical conditions (diabetes), per visit
S0618	Audiometry for hearing aid evaluation to determine the level and degree of hearing loss
S3850	Genetic testing for sickle cell anemia
S4990	Nicotine patches, legend

National T Codes (Codes T1000–T5999)

Code	Description
T1000	Private duty nursing, licensed, up to 15 minutes
T1013	Sign language or oral interpretive services, per 15 minutes
T1502	Administration of oral, intramuscular, and/or subcutaneous medication by health-care agency/professional, per visit
T2042	Hospice routine home care; per diem

Vision Services (Codes V2020–V2799)

Code	Description
V2020	Frames, purchases
V2219	Bifocal seg width over 28 mm
V2522	Contact lens, hydrophilic, bifocal, per lens
V2630	Anterior chamber intraocular lens

Hearing Services (Codes V5008–V5364)

Code	Description
V5008	Hearing screening
V5010	Assessment for hearing aid
V5362	Speech screening
V5363	Language screening

Many of the abbreviations listed in the HCPCS Level II book along with other commonly used abbreviations are in Tab 1. The Table of Drugs, National Coverage Determinations Manual, and National Average Payment can be reviewed in the HCPCS Level II book.

Modifiers (Appendix 1)

This table represents the most commonly used HCPCS modifiers. A complete listing can be found in the HCPCS book.

HCPCS	Description
AH	Clinical psychologist
AJ	Clinical social worker
AS	Assistant at surgery service
CC	Procedure code change
E1	Upper left eyelid
E2	Lower left eyelid
E3	Upper right eyelid
E4	Lower right eyelid
F1	Left hand, second digit
F2	Left hand, third digit
F3	Left hand, fourth digit
F4	Left hand, fifth digit
F5	Right hand, thumb
F6	Right hand, second digit
F7	Right hand, third digit
F8	Right hand, fourth digit
F9	Right hand, fifth digit
FA	Left hand, thumb
G9	Monitored anesthesia care (MAC) for at-risk patient
GC	Resident/teaching service

(Continued text on following page)

HCPCS	Description
GE	Resident/primary care exception applies
GV	Attending physician, not hospice
LT	Left side
PC	Professional courtesy
Q6	Locum tenens MD service
QS	Monitored anesthesia care (MAC)
QW	CLIA-waived test
QX	CRNA service with MD medical direction
QY	Medically directed CRNA
QZ	CRNA service without medical direction by MD
RT	Right side
SA	Nurse practitioner with physician
SB	Nurse midwife service
SG	ASC facility service
T1	Left foot, second digit
T2	Left foot, third digit
T3	Left foot, fourth digit
T4	Left foot, fifth digit
T5	Right foot, great toe
T6	Right foot, second digit
T7	Right foot, third digit
T8	Right foot, fourth digit
T9	Right foot, fifth digit
TA	Left foot, great toe
TC	Technical component

Facility Phone Numbers

Main number: _____
Laboratory: _____
Fax: _____
X-ray: _____
X-ray fax: _____
PT: _____
PT fax: _____
EKG/EEG: _____
EKG/EEG fax: _____
Outpatient scheduling: _____
Outpatient scheduling fax: _____
Emergency room: _____
Emergency room fax: _____
Operating room: _____
Operating room fax: _____
Admissions: _____
Admissions fax: _____
Billing office: _____
Billing office fax: _____
Medical records: _____
Medical records fax: _____
Medical staff office: _____
Medical staff office fax: _____
Office manager's home number: _____
Office manager's fax number: _____
Office manager's cell: _____
Other important numbers:
1. _____
2. _____
3. _____
4. _____

Frequently Called Offices

Dr. _____
Address: _____
Phone: _____
Fax: _____

Dr. _____
Address: _____
Phone: _____
Fax: _____

Terminology, Prefixes, Suffixes, Directional Terms, Abbreviations, Acronyms

The following listing of prefixes, suffixes, directional terms, general medical terms, and abbreviations can be used in identification of diseases, conditions, operations, etc., and is essential when coding and billing for services and procedures. All hospitals have their own individual accepted abbreviations list. It can be prudent to obtain this list and review it against these abbreviations.

Prefixes, Acronyms, Abbreviations

	Description
A	Without, away from
A/A	Automobile accident
AA	Acute appendicitis, acute asthma, African American, alcohol abuse, antiarrhythmic agent
AAA	Acute anxiety attack, abdominal aortic aneurysm
AAO	Awake, alert, oriented
AB	Abdominal, abortion, Ace bandage, antibody
AAO	Awake, alert, oriented to time, place, and person

ABG	Arterial blood gases
ABN	Advanced beneficiary notice
a.c.	Before meals
Acro	Extremities, top
AD	Advance directives
ADL	Activity of daily living
AF	Atrial fibrillation
ALS	Advanced life support
AMA	Against medical advice, American Medical Association
Ambi	Both
ANT	Anterior
Aniso	Unequal
ASC	Ambulatory surgery center
APAP	Acetaminophen
APC	Ambulatory Payment Classification
AS	Left ear
Ass.	Assessment
AU	Both ears
A-V	Arteriovenous
BC	Birth control
BE	Barium enema
Bi	Two
BID	Twice a day
Bld	Blood
BL	Blood
BM	Bowel movement
BP	Blood pressure
BS	Blood sugar, bowel sounds, breath sounds

(Continued text on following page)

	Description
Bx	Biopsy
C	Contact, concentration, canine, cup, with
CC	Chief complaint, commercial carriers
C&S	Culture and sensitivity
Ca	Cancer, calcium
cal	Calorie
Cap	Capacity
CBC	Complete blood count
CCI	Correct coding initiative
CCU	Coronary care unit
CHF	Congestive heart failure
Cir	Circumference
CM	Centimeter
CMN	Certificate of Medical Necessity
CMS	Centers for Medicare and Medicaid Services
COB	Coordination of benefits
COBRA	Consolidated Omnibus Reconciliation Act
COPD	Chronic obstructive pulmonary disease
CPAP	Continuous positive airway pressure
CPT	Current Procedural Terminology
CPR	Computerized patient record
CRF	Chronic renal failure
CRNA	Certified registered nurse anesthetist
CSW	Clinical social worker
CT	Computed tomography
Cu	Cubic
CXR	Chest x-ray
D	Day, date, dead, density, diarrhea, died, divorced, dose, duration, diameter

	Description
DAT	Diet as tolerated
DEC	Decease
Dec'd	deceased
DC	Decrease, discontinue
Deg	Degree
Dermo	Skin
Diplo	Double
Dist	Distal
DJD	Degenerative joint disease
DM	Diabetes mellitus
DME	Durable medical equipment
DNR	Do not resuscitate
DO	Doctor of Osteopathy
DOA	Dead on arrival
DOB	Date of birth
DOE	Dyspnea on exertion
DOS	Date of service
DPM	Doctor of Podiatric Medicine
DTR	Deep tendon reflex
Dx	Diagnosis
Dys	Bad, painful
Dur	duration
ED	Emergency department
EDI	Electronic data interchange
EEG	Electroencephalogram
ECG, EKG	Electrocardiogram
EENT	Eyes, ears, nose, throat

(Continued text on following page)

	Description
e.g.	For example
EMR	Electronic medical record
E&M	Evaluation and Management
EOB	Explanation of benefits
EOMB	Explanation of Medicare benefits
EPO	Exclusive provider organization
EPSDT	Early periodic screening, diagnosis, and treatment
ER	Emergency room
Erythro	Red
ETOH	Ethanol (alcohol)
Eu	Normal
Ext	Extended
F	Flexion, fluid, foot, from, frequency
Fld	Fluid
Ft	Foot
FTE	Full-time employee
F/u	Follow-up
FUO	Fever, unknown origin
G	Gram, gas, gravity, group
Ga	Gauge
GI	Gastrointestinal
gtt	drop
GU	Genitourinary
GYN	Gynecology
GR	Grain
GRP	Group
H	High, horizontal, human, hour, hundred

	Description
HA	Headache
HARPS	Heat, altered function, redness, pain, swelling
HCG	Human chorionic gonadotropin (pregnancy test)
HCPCS	Healthcare Common Procedural Coding System
HCT	Hematocrit
HEENT	Head, eyes, ears, nose, throat
HGB	Hemoglobin
HHA	Home health agency
HHS	Health and Human Services
HIPAA	Health Insurance Portability and Accountability Act
HOH	Hard of hearing
HPI	History of present illness
H&P	History and physical
HPSA	Health professional shortage area
HR	Hour, heart rate
Ht	Height
HTN	Hypertension
Hu	Human
Hypo	Hypodermic
Hetero	Different
Hex	Six
HMO	Health maintenance organization
Homo	Same
Hyper	High, increased
Hypo	Low, decreased
Hx	History

(Continued text on following page)

TOOLS

	Description
I	Inactive, increased, incontinent, initial, inspiration, insulin, intake, intensity, intermediate, iodine, iris, isotope
ICD-9-CM	International Classification of Disease, 9th Revision, Clinical Modification
ICF	Intermediate care facility
ICU	Intensive care unit
ID	Intradermal
I&D	Incision and drainage
IM	Intramuscular
IMP	Impression
INH	Inhalation
INS, Ins	Insulin, insurance
Int	Intermediate
Inter	Between
Intra	Inside
Ip	Interphalangeal
IPA	Individual practice association
IPO	Individual practice organization
Iso	Equal, same
IV	Intravenous
K	Potassium
KUB	Kidney, ureters, and bladder
J, jaund	Jaundice
JCAHO	Joint Commission for the Accreditation of Health Organization
L	Liter, length, left, long, longitudinal
L&D	Labor and delivery
LT	Left

	Description
Leuko	White
LFT	Liver function test
LLQ	Left lower quadrant
LOC	Loss of consciousness
LUQ	Left upper quadrant
LMP	Last menstrual period
LPN	Licensed practical nurse
M	By mouth, mass, mean, median, meter, minute, morphine, mucoid, murmur
MA	Medicaid
Mal	Poor
MC	Medicare
MCAL	Medicaid (California)
MCE	Medical care evaluation
MCM	Medicare Carriers Manual
MCP	Monthly capitation payment
MD	Median, Medical Doctor, Medicaid
MDM	Medical decision-making
MSP	Medicare secondary payor
Megalo	Large
Melano	Black, dark
MH	Maternal history, mental health
MHx	Medical history
Min	Minute
MLP	Midlevel provider
mm	millimeter
Mono	One
MRA	Magnetic resonance angiography

(Continued text on following page)

	Description
MRI	Magnetic resonance imaging
MVA	Motor vehicle accident
N	Nasal, nerve, night, normal, number
NA	Sodium
NAD	No acute distress
NAIC	National Association of Insurance Commissioners
Nas	Nasal
NEC	Not elsewhere classified
NH	Nursing home
NKA	No known allergies
NKDA	No known drug allergies
ng	Nasogastric
NL	Normal
No	Number
Noc	At night
NOS	Not otherwise specified
NP	Nurse practitioner
NPI	National provider identifier
NSR	Normal sinus rhythm
N/V	Nausea/vomiting
N/V/D	Nausea,/vomiting/diarrhea
OB	Obstetrics
OD	Daily
OMT	Osteopathic manipulation therapy
OPL	Other party liability
OPPS	Outpatient Prospective Payment System
os	Mouth
OT	Occupational therapy

	Description
OTC	Over-the-counter
ou	Both eyes
P	Page, after (post), para, partial, peripheral, phosphate, pint, pupil, pressure, pulse
PA	Physician assistant
PC	Professional courtesy, professional component
p.c.	After meals
PCP	Primary care physician
PE	Physical exam
PERLA	Pupils equal and reactive to light accommodation
PFSH	Past, family, social history
PIN	Physician identification number
PMH	Past medical history
PMPM	Per member per month
PMPY	Per member per year
po	By mouth
Polio	Gray
POS	Point of service, place of service
PPO	Preferred provider organization
pr	Through the rectum
PRN	As needed
PRO	Peer review organization
PSA	Prostate specific antigen
PSH	Past surgical history
pt	pint
PT	Physical therapy, prothrombin time, patient
PTT	Partial thromboplastin
PVC	Premature ventricular complex

(Continued text on following page)

	Description
Q	Each, every, four (quad), quantity, quart, quarter, volume
qd	Every day
qh	Every hour
qod	Every other day
QID	Four times a day
Qty	Quantity
Qt	Quart
Qr	Quarter
Quad	Four
R	Respirations, radius, round
RA	Remittance advice
RBC	Red blood count
RBRVS	Resource-based relative value study
R&C	Reasonable and customary
RICE	Rest, ice, compression, elevation
RLQ	Right lower quadrant
R/O	Rule-out
ROE	Roentgen
ROM	Range of motion
ROS	Review of systems
RN	Registered nurse
RUQ	Right upper quadrant
Rx	Prescription
S	Distance, label, left, second, section, sensation, series, sign, steady state
s	without
sc, sq	Subcutaneous

	Description
Sec, SEC	Second, section
Ser	Series
Sex	Six
SL	Sublingual
SNF	Skilled nursing facility
SOB	Shortness of breath
Sol	Solution
SHx	Surgical history
STAT	Immediately
Sx	Symptoms
SZ	Seizure
T	Temperature, duration, life, teaspoonful, temporal, terminal, tertiary, test, time, ton
Tabs	Tablets
T&C	Type and cross
TC	Technical component
TCC	Transitional care center
Term/TRML	Terminal
Ter	Tertiary
TID	Three times per day
TPA	Third-party administrator
TPL	Third-party liability
TM	Temporomandibular
TPN	Total parenteral nutrition
TPP	Third-party payor
TPR	Temperature, pulse, and respiration
Tri	Three
TQM	Total quality management

(Continued text on following page)

	Description
Tx	Treatment
UA	Urinalysis, uric acid
UCR	Usual, customary, and reasonable
Uni	One
UPIN	Unique physician identification number
URI	Upper respiratory infection
US	Ultrasound
UTI	Urinary tract infection
V	Vein, velocity, venous, versus, virus
VB	Venous blood
Vir	Virus
VIT	Vitamin
VS	Vital signs
W	Watt, week, weight, white, widowed, wife
WC, WComp	Workers Compensation
WH	White
WNL	Within normal limits
wk	Week
Wt	Weight
Xantho	yellow
Y	Year, yield
Yr	Year

Suffixes	
	Description
-algia	Pain
-asthenia	Weakness

	Description
-centesis	Removal of fluid through a puncture into a body cavity
-ectomy	Excision/surgical removal
-emia	Blood
-iasis	Condition of
-itis	Inflammation
-lysis	Destruction
-lytic	Breakdown
-megaly	Enlarged
-oid	Like
-oma	Tumor
-opathy	Disease of
-opexy	Surgical fixation
-oplasty	Surgical repair
-otripsy	Crushing, destroying
-orrhagia	Hemorrhage
-orrhaphy	Surgical repair/suture
-orrhea	Discharge
-osis	Abnormal condition of
-ostomy	Permanent opening (new)
-otomy	Incision
-orrhaphy	Suture
-paresis	Weakness
-plasia	Growth
-plegia	paralysis
-pnea	Breathing
-rrahgia	Excessive flow
-rrhea	Flowing
-rrhexis	Rupture

(Continued text on following page)

Directions	
Word	**Description**
Anterior	At/near the front surface of the body
Distal	Farthest from the center
Inferior	Below
Lateral	Side
Medial	Middle
Posterior	At/near the back surface of the body
Prone	Face down/palm down
Proximal	Nearest to the center
Superior	Above
Supine	Face up/palm up

Body Planes	
Word	**Description**
Coronal	Vertical body plane, divides the body into front and back sections
Sagittal	Vertical body plane, divides the body into equal right and left sides
Transverse	Horizontal body plane, divides the body into top and bottom sections

State Medicare Carriers

State	Medicare Carrier
Alabama	Blue Cross/Blue Shield of Alabama PO Box 830139, Birmingham, AL 35283-0139 Phone: 205-988-2100; Fax: 205-981-4841
Alaska	Noridian Mutual Insurance Company 4305 13th Ave SW Fargo, ND 58103 Phone: 701-282-1100; Fax: 701-282-1002
Arizona	Noridian Mutual Insurance Company 4305 13th Ave SW Fargo, ND 58103 Phone: 701-282-1100; Fax: 701-282-1002
Arkansas	Arkansas Blue Cross/Blue Shield, A Mutual Insurance Company 601 Gaines St Little Rock, AR 72201 Phone: 501-378-2000; Fax: 501-378-2804
California	National Heritage Insurance Company 402 Otterson Drive Chico, CA 95928 Phone: 530-896-7400; Fax: 530-896-7182
Colorado	Noridian Mutual Insurance Company 4305 13th Ave SW Fargo, ND 58103 Phone: 701-282-1100; Fax: 701-282-1002
Connecticut	Trailblazer Health Enterprises, LLC PO Box 660156 Dallas, TX 75266 Phone: 972-766-6900; Fax: 972-766-1765

(Continued text on following page)

State Medicare Carriers *(Continued)*

State	Medicare Carrier
Delaware	Trailblazer Health Enterprises, LLC PO Box 660156 Dallas, TX 75266 Phone: 972-766-6900; Fax: 972-766-1765
District of Columbia	Trailblazer Health Enterprises, LLC PO Box 660156 Dallas, TX 75266 Phone: 972-766-6900; Fax: 972-766-1765
Florida	Blue Cross/Blue Shield of Florida, Inc. 532 Riverside Ave Jacksonville, FL 32202 Phone: 904-791-6111; Fax: 904-905-6020
Georgia	Blue Cross/Blue Shield of Alabama PO Box 830139, Birmingham, AL 35283-0139 Phone: 205-988-2100; Fax: 205-981-4841
Hawaii	Noridian Mutual Insurance Company 4305 13th Ave SW Fargo, ND 58103 Phone: 701-282-1100; Fax: 701-282-1002
Idaho	Connecticut General Life Insurance Company Hartford, CT 06152 Phone: 615-782-4576 Fax: 615-244-6242
Illinois	National Heritage Insurance Company 402 Otterson Drive Chico, CA 95928 Phone: 530-896-7400; Fax: 530-896-7182
Indiana	AdminaStar Federal, Inc. 8115 Knue Road Indianapolis, IN 46250 Phone: 317-841-4400; Fax: 317-841-4691

State Medicare Carriers *(Continued)*

State	Medicare Carrier
Iowa	Noridian Mutual Insurance Company 4305 13th Ave SW Fargo, ND 58103 Phone: 701-282-1100; Fax: 701-282-1002
Kansas	Blue Cross/Blue Shield of Kansas, Inc. 1133 Topeka Ave Topeka, KS 66629 Phone: 785-291-7000; Fax: 785-291-7098
Kentucky	AdminaStar Federal, Inc. 8115 Knue Road Indianapolis, IN 46250 Phone: 317-841-4400; Fax: 317-841-4691
Louisiana	Arkansas Blue Cross/Blue Shield, A Mutual Insurance Company 601 Gaines St Little Rock, AR 72201 Phone: 501-378-2000; Fax: 501-378-2804
Maine	National Heritage Insurance Company 402 Otterson Drive Chico, CA 95928 Phone: 530-896-7400; Fax: 530-896-7182
Maryland	Trailblazer Health Enterprises, LLC PO Box 660156 Dallas, TX 75266 Phone: 972-766-6900; Fax: 972-766-1765
Massachusetts	National Heritage Insurance Company 402 Otterson Drive Chico, CA 95928 Phone: 530-896-7400; Fax: 530-896-7182

(Continued text on following page)

State Medicare Carriers *(Continued)*

State	Medicare Carrier
Michigan	National Heritage Insurance Company 402 Otterson Drive Chico, CA 95928 Phone: 530-896-7400; Fax: 530-896-7182
Minnesota	Wisconsin Physicians Insurance Corporation PO Box 8190 Madison, WI 53708 Phone: 608-221-4711; Fax: 608-223-3614
Mississippi	Wisconsin Physicians Insurance Corporation PO Box 8190 Madison, WI 53708 Phone: 608-221-4711; Fax: 608-223-3614
Missouri	Blue Cross/Blue Shield of Kansas, Inc. 1133 Topeka Ave Topeka, KS 66629 Phone: 785-291-7000; Fax: 785-291-7098
Montana	Blue Cross/Blue Shield of Montana, Inc. PO Box 4310, 340 N. Last Chance Gulch Helena, MT 59604 Phone: 406-444-8350; Fax: 406-442-9968
Nebraska	Blue Cross/Blue Shield of Kansas, Inc. 1133 Topeka Ave Topeka, KS 66629 Phone: 785-291-7000; Fax: 785-291-7098
Nevada	Noridian Mutual Insurance Company 4305 13th Ave SW Fargo, ND 58103 Phone: 701-282-1100; Fax: 701-282-1002

State Medicare Carriers *(Continued)*

State	Medicare Carrier
New Hampshire	National Heritage Insurance Company 402 Otterson Drive Chico, CA 95928 Phone: 530-896-7400; Fax: 530-896-7182
New Jersey	Highmark, Inc C/O HGSAdministrators PO Box 8900065 Camp Hill, PA 17089 Phone: 717-763-3151; Fax: 717-975-7045
New Mexico	Arkansas Blue Cross/Blue Shield, A Mutual Insurance Company 601 Gaines St Little Rock, AR 72201 Phone: 501-378-2000; Fax: 501-378-2804
New York	
Counties of Bronx Columbia, Delaware, Duchess, Greene, Kings, Nassau, New York, Orange, Putnam, Richmond, Rockland, Suffolk, Sullivan, Ulster, Westchester	Empire Medicare Services PO Box 2280 Peekskill, NY 10566 Phone: 866-837-0241; Fax: 866-709-1905
Queens	Group Health Incorporated 88 West End Avenue New York, NY 10023 Phone: 212-721-1300; Fax: 212-721-0580

(Continued text on following page)

TOOLS

State Medicare Carriers *(Continued)*

State	Medicare Carrier
Virginia	Trailblazer Health Enterprises, LLC PO Box 660156 Dallas, TX 75266 Phone: 972-766-6900; Fax: 972-766-1765
Washington	Noridian Mutual Insurance Company 4305 13th Ave SW Fargo, ND 58103 Phone: 701-282-1100; Fax: 701-282-1002
West Virginia	Nationwide Mutual Insurance Company PO Box 16788 Columbus, OH 43216 Phone: 614-249-7111; Fax: 614-249-3732
Wisconsin	Wisconsin Physicians Insurance Corporation PO Box 8190 Madison, WI 53708 Phone: 608-221-4711; Fax: 608-223-3614
Wyoming	Noridian Mutual Insurance Company 4305 13th Ave SW Fargo, ND 58103 Phone: 701-282-1100; Fax: 701-282-1002
Puerto Rico	Triple-S, Inc PO Box 71391 San Juan, PR 00936 Phone: 787-749-4080; Fax: 787-749-4092
Virgin Islands	Triple-S, Inc PO Box 71391 San Juan, PR 00936 Phone: 787-749-4080; Fax: 787-749-4092

Web Sites of Interest

Organization/Association	Web Site
Center for Medicare and Medicaid Services	www.cms.gov
Code of Federal Regulations	www.access.gpo.gov/nara/cfr
Department of Health and Human Services	www.dhhs.gov
Government Printing Office	www.access.gpo.gov
Local Carrier Info-Medicare	www.cms.gov/regions/default.htm
Office of Inspector General Workplan	www.hhs.gov/progorg/wrkpln/index.html
Office of Inspector General Compliance Plans	www.dhhs.gov/progorg/oig
American Academy of Professional Coders	www.aapcnatl.org
American College of Healthcare Executives	www.ache.org
American Health Management Information Association	www.ahima.org
Healthcare Financial Management Association	www.hfma.org
Medical Group Management Association	www.mgma.com
Center for Healthcare Information Management	www.chim.org
Human Anatomy	www.mnsu.edu/emuseum/biology/humananatomy/index.shtml
Medical Abbreviations	www.pharma-lexicon.com/

Index

Davis's Notes

Your Handheld Clinical Companions

e vital clinical information you need!

PAA-supportive, wipe-free, waterproof,
sable patient assessment tools and worksheets
rtable, indispensable, pocket-sized tools for safe
d effective health care delivery

ing Notes: Medical Insurance Pocket Guide

ides students and practicing Medical Assistants
an easy-to-understand medical billing and
ng reference. Formatted in text, tables, and
s to help users quickly and accurately find
rmation for immediate use.

Coding Notes—Coding and billing made easy!

Look for our other Davis's Notes titles

RNotes® • MedSurg Notes • NutriNotes • MedNotes • LPN Notes
MA Notes: Medical Assistant's Pocket Guide
IV Therapy Notes: Nurse's Clinical Pocket Guide
LabNotes: Guide to Lab & Diagnostic Tests
ECG Notes: Interpretation and Management Guide

Visit us at www.FADavis.com

F.A. Davis Company
Independent Publishers Since 1879

ISBN 10: 0-8036-1493-4
ISBN 13: 978-0-8036-1493-2

9 780803 614932

Inches Centimeters